THIS KETO DIET

Journal Belongs To:

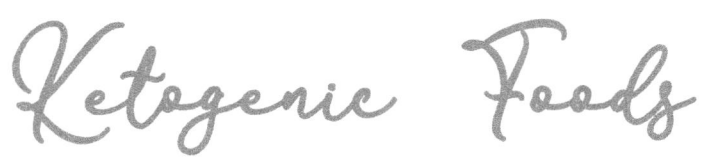

Ketogenic Foods

MEATS

Beef
Sausage
Bacon
Lamb
Pork
Veal
Chicken/Turkey
Eggs

VEGGIES

Avocado
Asparagus
Argula
Broccoli
Cauliflower
Brussel Sprouts
Cabbage
Celery

VEGGIES

Cucumber
Chards
Bell Peppers
Green Beans
Collards
Mushrooms
Spinach
Olives

FRUITS

Blackberries
Cranberries
Blueberries
Lemon
Lime
Raspberries
Strawberries
Plantains (paleo)

DAIRY

Cheese (all kinds)
Sour Cream
Cream Cheese
Heavy Cream
Greek Yogurt
Almond Milk
Cashew Milk
Coconut Cream

CONDIMENTS

Balsamic Vinegar
Beef/Chicken Broth
Bonito Flakes
Tartar Sauce (keto)
Dijon Mustard
Mayo
Low Sugar Ketchup
Pickles

OILS & FATS

Avocado Oil
Butter
Coconut Butter
Duck Fat
Lard/Ghee
Nut Oils
Olive Oil
Pork Rinds

HERBS & SPICES

Garlic
Salt & Pepper
Oregano
Paprika
Cumin
Chili Pepper
Basil
Ginger

BAKING

Almond Flour
Almond Meal
Cashew Flour
Oat Fiber
Psyllium Husk
Whey Protein
Flax meal
Hazelnut Flour

FISH/SEAFOOD

Anchovy
Haddock / Cod
Halibut
Crab/Lobster
Mackerel
Salmon
Tuna
Red Snapper

DRINKS

Diet Soda (moderation)
Coffee
Tea
Gatorade Zero
Protein Shake
Club Soda
Broth
Coconut Water

MISC.

Canned Tuna
Pesto
Soy Sauce
Aioli
Béarnaise
Vinaigrette
Hot Sauce
Guacamole

NOTES:

Macro Quick Reference

MACRO TRACKER

QTY	TYPE	PROTEIN	FAT	CARBS	CALS	NOTES

Low Carb Grocery Ideas

FRESH PRODUCE

Asparagus	Cauliflower	Onions
Avocado	Celery	Radishes
Bell Peppers	Cucumber	Salad Mix
Berries	Eggplant	Squash
Broccoli	Fennel	Tomatoes
Brussel Sprouts	Garlic	Bok Choi
Cabbage	Green Beans	Chives
Carrots	Mushrooms	Spinach

MEAT AND SEAFOOD

Bacon	Lamb	Fish
Beef	Pork	Crab
Bison	Rotisserie Chicken	Lobster
Chicken	Sausage	Scallops
Deli meat	Turkey	Shrimp
Ground Beef / Ground Turkey	Oyster	Mussels

DAIRY PRODUCTS

Butter	Eggs	Sour Cream
Cheese	Greek Yogurt, full fat	Ghee
Cream Cheese	Heavy Whipping Cream	Mayo

PANTRY ITEMS

Avocado oil	Tea/Coffee	Moon Cheese
Beef Jerky	Pork Rinds	Low Carb Protein Bars
Bone Broth	Mayonnaise	All Natural Peanut Butter
Tuna, Salmon (canned)	Low Carb Salad Dressing	Stevia
Coconut Butter	Olive oil, extra virgin	Almonds
Coconut Oil	Olives	Spices
Almond Milk	Sweeteners	Almond Flour

FROZEN / OTHER

Low Carb Shopping List

FRESH PRODUCE

MEAT AND SEAFOOD

DAIRY PRODUCTS

PANTRY ITEMS

FROZEN / OTHER

Keto 15 Task Challenge

1

CREATE A KETO
JOURNAL AND DOCUMENT
YOUR PROGRESS

COMPLETED

2

CHOOSE 7 KETO FRIENDLY
RECIPES TO TRY

COMPLETED

3

CREATE A WEEKLY
MEAL PLANNER

COMPLETED

4

LOG EVERYTHING YOU EAT
IN A WEIGHT LOSS APP

COMPLETED

5

PURCHASE A FOOD SCALE
AND SPIRALIZER

COMPLETED

6

TRY BULLET PROOF
COFFEE

COMPLETED

7

WEIGH YOURSELF
EVERY WEEK

COMPLETED

8

GO ALCOHOL FREE FOR
ONE WEEK

COMPLETED

9

TRY A 12-HOUR
INTERMITTENT FAST

COMPLETED

10

CHECK AND LOG YOUR
BODY MEASUREMENTS

COMPLETED

11

LIST ALL THE REASONS WHY
KETO WILL WORK FOR YOU

COMPLETED

12

LEARN TO MAKE FAT BOMBS

COMPLETED

13

MONITOR YOUR
WATER INTAKE

COMPLETED

14

INCREASE YOUR HEALTHY
FAT INTAKE

COMPLETED

15

TEST KETONE LEVELS
USING STRIPS

COMPLETED

INTERMITTENT *Fasting Log*

WEEK OF:

	START TIME	END TIME	TOTAL FAST HRS
M	:	:	:
T	:	:	:
W	:	:	:
T	:	:	:
F	:	:	:
S	:	:	:
S	:	:	:

WEEK OF:

	START TIME	END TIME	TOTAL FAST HRS
M	:	:	:
T	:	:	:
W	:	:	:
T	:	:	:
F	:	:	:
S	:	:	:
S	:	:	:

WEEK OF:

	START TIME	END TIME	TOTAL FAST HRS
M	:	:	:
T	:	:	:
W	:	:	:
T	:	:	:
F	:	:	:
S	:	:	:
S	:	:	:

WEEK OF:

	START TIME	END TIME	TOTAL FAST HRS
M	:	:	:
T	:	:	:
W	:	:	:
T	:	:	:
F	:	:	:
S	:	:	:
S	:	:	:

WEEK OF:

	START TIME	END TIME	TOTAL FAST HRS
M	:	:	:
T	:	:	:
W	:	:	:
T	:	:	:
F	:	:	:
S	:	:	:
S	:	:	:

WEEK OF:

	START TIME	END TIME	TOTAL FAST HRS
M	:	:	:
T	:	:	:
W	:	:	:
T	:	:	:
F	:	:	:
S	:	:	:
S	:	:	:

MILESTONES & ACCOMPLISHMENTS

NOTES & REFLECTIONS

KETO GO TO *Meals*

BREAKFAST	LUNCH	DINNER	SNACKS
BREAKFAST	LUNCH	DINNER	SNACKS
BREAKFAST	LUNCH	DINNER	SNACKS
BREAKFAST	LUNCH	DINNER	SNACKS
BREAKFAST	LUNCH	DINNER	SNACKS
BREAKFAST	LUNCH	DINNER	SNACKS
BREAKFAST	LUNCH	DINNER	SNACKS

KETO BEFORE & After

WEIGHT

BMI

BODY FAT

MUSCLE

CHEST

WAIST

HIPS

THIGHS

CALF

BICEP

OTHER :

OTHER :

WEIGHT

BMI

BODY FAT

MUSCLE

CHEST

WAIST

HIPS

THIGHS

CALF

BICEP

OTHER :

OTHER :

WEIGHT LOSS *Tracker*

MONTHLY GOAL

DATE:

	CHEST				
	WAIST				
	SHOULDERS				
	UPPER ARM				
	FOREARM				
	CALF				
	WEIGHT				
TOTAL WEIGHT LOSS >>					

WEIGHT LOSS *Tracker*

MONTHLY GOAL

DATE:

	BUST				
	WAIST				
	HIPS				
	BICEP				
	THIGH				
	CALF				
	WEIGHT				
TOTAL WEIGHT LOSS >>					

100 Days of Keto

STARTING WEIGHT: **DAY 100 WEIGHT:**

1	2	3	4	5	6	7	8	9	10	LBS LOST: INCHES LOST:
11	12	13	14	15	16	17	18	19	20	LBS LOST: INCHES LOST:
21	22	23	24	25	26	27	28	29	30	LBS LOST: INCHES LOST:
31	32	33	34	35	36	37	38	39	40	LBS LOST: INCHES LOST:
41	42	43	44	45	46	47	48	49	50	LBS LOST: INCHES LOST:
51	52	53	54	55	56	57	58	59	60	LBS LOST: INCHES LOST:
61	62	63	64	65	66	67	68	69	70	LBS LOST: INCHES LOST:
71	72	73	74	75	76	77	78	79	80	LBS LOST: INCHES LOST:
81	82	83	84	85	86	87	88	89	90	LBS LOST: INCHES LOST:
91	92	93	94	95	96	97	98	99	100	LBS LOST: INCHES LOST:

TOTAL WEIGHT LOST: **TOTAL INCHES LOST:**

NOTES & REFLECTIONS:

MEAL 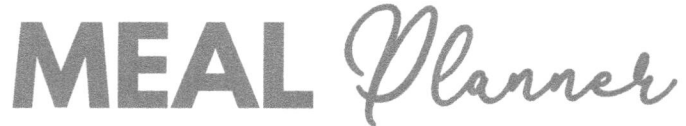 Planner

WEEK OF

GROCERY LIST

MON

TUES

WED

THUR

FRI

SAT

SUN

Weekly Meal Planner

Week of: _____

	Breakfast	Lunch	Dinner	Snack	Other
Monday	TOTAL Carbs Fat Protein Cals	TOTAL Carbs Fat Protein Cals	TOTAL Carbs Fat Protein Cals	TOTAL Carbs Fat Protein Cals	TOTAL Carbs Fat Protein Cals
Tuesday	TOTAL Carbs Fat Protein Cals	TOTAL Carbs Fat Protein Cals	TOTAL Carbs Fat Protein Cals	TOTAL Carbs Fat Protein Cals	TOTAL Carbs Fat Protein Cals
Wednesday	TOTAL Carbs Fat Protein Cals	TOTAL Carbs Fat Protein Cals	TOTAL Carbs Fat Protein Cals	TOTAL Carbs Fat Protein Cals	TOTAL Carbs Fat Protein Cals
Thursday	TOTAL Carbs Fat Protein Cals	TOTAL Carbs Fat Protein Cals	TOTAL Carbs Fat Protein Cals	TOTAL Carbs Fat Protein Cals	TOTAL Carbs Fat Protein Cals
Friday	TOTAL Carbs Fat Protein Cals	TOTAL Carbs Fat Protein Cals	TOTAL Carbs Fat Protein Cals	TOTAL Carbs Fat Protein Cals	TOTAL Carbs Fat Protein Cals
Saturday	TOTAL Carbs Fat Protein Cals	TOTAL Carbs Fat Protein Cals	TOTAL Carbs Fat Protein Cals	TOTAL Carbs Fat Protein Cals	TOTAL Carbs Fat Protein Cals
Sunday	TOTAL Carbs Fat Protein Cals	TOTAL Carbs Fat Protein Cals	TOTAL Carbs Fat Protein Cals	TOTAL Carbs Fat Protein Cals	TOTAL Carbs Fat Protein Cals

MY PROGRESS *Tracker*

SLEEP TRACKER:

DATE _____

 RISE: _____

 BEDTIME: _____

 SLEEP (HRS): _____

NOTES FOR THE DAY

_____

_____

_____

IN A STATE OF KETOSIS?

YES   NO   UNSURE

WATER INTAKE TRACKER

EXERCISE / WORKOUT ROUTINE

DAILY ENERGY LEVEL		
HIGH	**MEDIUM**	**LOW**

BREAKFAST

FAT: CARBS: PROTEIN: CALORIES:

LUNCH

FAT: CARBS: PROTEIN: CALORIES:

DINNER

FAT: CARBS: PROTEIN: CALORIES:

SNACKS

FAT: CARBS: PROTEIN: CALORIES:

TOP 6 PRIORITIES OF THE DAY

END OF THE DAY TOTAL OVERVIEW

CARBS	FAT	PROTEIN	CALORIES
☐	☐	☐	☐

MY PROGRESS *Tracker*

SLEEP TRACKER:

 RISE:

 BEDTIME:

DATE _____

 SLEEP (HRS):

NOTES FOR THE DAY

_____

_____

_____

IN A STATE OF KETOSIS?

YES   NO   UNSURE

WATER INTAKE TRACKER

EXERCISE / WORKOUT ROUTINE

DAILY ENERGY LEVEL		
HIGH	**MEDIUM**	**LOW**

BREAKFAST

FAT: CARBS: PROTEIN: CALORIES:

LUNCH

FAT: CARBS: PROTEIN: CALORIES:

DINNER

FAT: CARBS: PROTEIN: CALORIES:

SNACKS

FAT: CARBS: PROTEIN: CALORIES:

TOP 6 PRIORITIES OF THE DAY

END OF THE DAY TOTAL OVERVIEW

CARBS	FAT	PROTEIN	CALORIES

MY PROGRESS *Tracker*

SLEEP TRACKER:

 RISE: [_____]   BEDTIME: [_____]   SLEEP (HRS): [_____]

NOTES FOR THE DAY

_____

_____

IN A STATE OF KETOSIS?

YES   NO   UNSURE

WATER INTAKE TRACKER

EXERCISE / WORKOUT ROUTINE

DAILY ENERGY LEVEL		
HIGH	**MEDIUM**	**LOW**

BREAKFAST

FAT: CARBS: PROTEIN: CALORIES:

LUNCH

FAT: CARBS: PROTEIN: CALORIES:

DINNER

FAT: CARBS: PROTEIN: CALORIES:

SNACKS

FAT: CARBS: PROTEIN: CALORIES:

TOP 6 PRIORITIES OF THE DAY

END OF THE DAY TOTAL OVERVIEW

CARBS   FAT   PROTEIN   CALORIES

[   ]   [   ]   [   ]   [   ]

MY PROGRESS *Tracker*

SLEEP TRACKER:

DATE _____

 RISE: | BEDTIME: | SLEEP (HRS):

NOTES FOR THE DAY

_____

_____

_____

IN A STATE OF KETOSIS?

YES   NO   UNSURE

WATER INTAKE TRACKER

EXERCISE / WORKOUT ROUTINE

DAILY ENERGY LEVEL		
HIGH	**MEDIUM**	**LOW**

BREAKFAST

FAT: CARBS: PROTEIN: CALORIES:

LUNCH

FAT: CARBS: PROTEIN: CALORIES:

DINNER

FAT: CARBS: PROTEIN: CALORIES:

SNACKS

FAT: CARBS: PROTEIN: CALORIES:

TOP 6 PRIORITIES OF THE DAY

END OF THE DAY TOTAL OVERVIEW

CARBS	FAT	PROTEIN	CALORIES

MY PROGRESS *Tracker*

SLEEP TRACKER:

DATE _____

 RISE: _____   BEDTIME: _____   SLEEP (HRS): _____

NOTES FOR THE DAY

_____

_____

_____

IN A STATE OF KETOSIS?

YES   NO   UNSURE

WATER INTAKE TRACKER

EXERCISE / WORKOUT ROUTINE

DAILY ENERGY LEVEL		
HIGH	**MEDIUM**	**LOW**

BREAKFAST

FAT: CARBS: PROTEIN: CALORIES:

LUNCH

FAT: CARBS: PROTEIN: CALORIES:

DINNER

FAT: CARBS: PROTEIN: CALORIES:

SNACKS

FAT: CARBS: PROTEIN: CALORIES:

TOP 6 PRIORITIES OF THE DAY

END OF THE DAY TOTAL OVERVIEW

CARBS	FAT	PROTEIN	CALORIES

MY PROGRESS *Tracker*

SLEEP TRACKER:

DATE _____

 RISE: _____   BEDTIME: _____   SLEEP (HRS): _____

NOTES FOR THE DAY

_____

_____

_____

IN A STATE OF KETOSIS?

YES   NO   UNSURE

WATER INTAKE TRACKER

EXERCISE / WORKOUT ROUTINE

DAILY ENERGY LEVEL		
HIGH	**MEDIUM**	**LOW**

BREAKFAST

FAT: CARBS: PROTEIN: CALORIES:

LUNCH

FAT: CARBS: PROTEIN: CALORIES:

DINNER

FAT: CARBS: PROTEIN: CALORIES:

SNACKS

FAT: CARBS: PROTEIN: CALORIES:

TOP 6 PRIORITIES OF THE DAY

END OF THE DAY TOTAL OVERVIEW

CARBS	FAT	PROTEIN	CALORIES

MY PROGRESS *Tracker*

SLEEP TRACKER:

DATE _____

 RISE: _____   BEDTIME: _____   SLEEP (HRS): _____

NOTES FOR THE DAY

_____

_____

_____

IN A STATE OF KETOSIS?

YES   NO   UNSURE

WATER INTAKE TRACKER

EXERCISE / WORKOUT ROUTINE

DAILY ENERGY LEVEL		
HIGH	**MEDIUM**	**LOW**

BREAKFAST

FAT: CARBS: PROTEIN: CALORIES:

LUNCH

FAT: CARBS: PROTEIN: CALORIES:

DINNER

FAT: CARBS: PROTEIN: CALORIES:

SNACKS

FAT: CARBS: PROTEIN: CALORIES:

TOP 6 PRIORITIES OF THE DAY

END OF THE DAY TOTAL OVERVIEW

CARBS	FAT	PROTEIN	CALORIES
	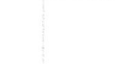		

MEAL *Planner*

GROCERY LIST

MON

TUES

WED

THUR

FRI

SAT

SUN

Weekly Meal Planner

Week of: _____

	Breakfast	Lunch	Dinner	Snack	Other
Monday	TOTAL Carbs Fat Protein Cals	TOTAL Carbs Fat Protein Cals	TOTAL Carbs Fat Protein Cals	TOTAL Carbs Fat Protein Cals	TOTAL Carbs Fat Protein Cals
Tuesday	TOTAL Carbs Fat Protein Cals	TOTAL Carbs Fat Protein Cals	TOTAL Carbs Fat Protein Cals	TOTAL Carbs Fat Protein Cals	TOTAL Carbs Fat Protein Cals
Wednesday	TOTAL Carbs Fat Protein Cals	TOTAL Carbs Fat Protein Cals	TOTAL Carbs Fat Protein Cals	TOTAL Carbs Fat Protein Cals	TOTAL Carbs Fat Protein Cals
Thursday	TOTAL Carbs Fat Protein Cals	TOTAL Carbs Fat Protein Cals	TOTAL Carbs Fat Protein Cals	TOTAL Carbs Fat Protein Cals	TOTAL Carbs Fat Protein Cals
Friday	TOTAL Carbs Fat Protein Cals	TOTAL Carbs Fat Protein Cals	TOTAL Carbs Fat Protein Cals	TOTAL Carbs Fat Protein Cals	TOTAL Carbs Fat Protein Cals
Saturday	TOTAL Carbs Fat Protein Cals	TOTAL Carbs Fat Protein Cals	TOTAL Carbs Fat Protein Cals	TOTAL Carbs Fat Protein Cals	TOTAL Carbs Fat Protein Cals
Sunday	TOTAL Carbs Fat Protein Cals	TOTAL Carbs Fat Protein Cals	TOTAL Carbs Fat Protein Cals	TOTAL Carbs Fat Protein Cals	TOTAL Carbs Fat Protein Cals

MY PROGRESS *Tracker*

SLEEP TRACKER:

DATE _____

 RISE: _____

 BEDTIME: _____

 SLEEP (HRS): _____

NOTES FOR THE DAY

_____

_____

IN A STATE OF KETOSIS?

YES   NO   UNSURE

WATER INTAKE TRACKER

EXERCISE / WORKOUT ROUTINE

DAILY ENERGY LEVEL		
HIGH	**MEDIUM**	**LOW**

BREAKFAST

FAT: CARBS: PROTEIN: CALORIES:

LUNCH

FAT: CARBS: PROTEIN: CALORIES:

DINNER

FAT: CARBS: PROTEIN: CALORIES:

SNACKS

FAT: CARBS: PROTEIN: CALORIES:

TOP 6 PRIORITIES OF THE DAY

END OF THE DAY TOTAL OVERVIEW

CARBS	FAT	PROTEIN	CALORIES

MY PROGRESS *Tracker*

SLEEP TRACKER:

DATE _____

 RISE: | BEDTIME: | SLEEP (HRS):

NOTES FOR THE DAY

_____
_____
_____

IN A STATE OF KETOSIS?

YES   NO   UNSURE

WATER INTAKE TRACKER

EXERCISE / WORKOUT ROUTINE

DAILY ENERGY LEVEL		
HIGH	**MEDIUM**	**LOW**

BREAKFAST

FAT: CARBS: PROTEIN: CALORIES:

LUNCH

FAT: CARBS: PROTEIN: CALORIES:

DINNER

FAT: CARBS: PROTEIN: CALORIES:

SNACKS

FAT: CARBS: PROTEIN: CALORIES:

TOP 6 PRIORITIES OF THE DAY

END OF THE DAY TOTAL OVERVIEW

CARBS   FAT   PROTEIN   CALORIES

  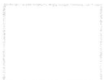 

MY PROGRESS *Tracker*

SLEEP TRACKER:

DATE _____

 RISE: _____   BEDTIME: _____   SLEEP (HRS): _____

NOTES FOR THE DAY

_____

_____

_____

IN A STATE OF KETOSIS?

YES   NO   UNSURE

WATER INTAKE TRACKER

EXERCISE / WORKOUT ROUTINE

DAILY ENERGY LEVEL		
HIGH	**MEDIUM**	**LOW**

BREAKFAST

FAT: CARBS: PROTEIN: CALORIES:

LUNCH

FAT: CARBS: PROTEIN: CALORIES:

DINNER

FAT: CARBS: PROTEIN: CALORIES:

SNACKS

FAT: CARBS: PROTEIN: CALORIES:

TOP 6 PRIORITIES OF THE DAY

END OF THE DAY TOTAL OVERVIEW

CARBS	FAT	PROTEIN	CALORIES

MY PROGRESS *Tracker*

SLEEP TRACKER:

DATE _____

 RISE: _____   BEDTIME: _____   SLEEP (HRS): _____

NOTES FOR THE DAY

_____

_____

_____

IN A STATE OF KETOSIS?

YES   NO   UNSURE

WATER INTAKE TRACKER

EXERCISE / WORKOUT ROUTINE

DAILY ENERGY LEVEL		
HIGH	**MEDIUM**	**LOW**

BREAKFAST

FAT: CARBS: PROTEIN: CALORIES:

LUNCH

FAT: CARBS: PROTEIN: CALORIES:

DINNER

FAT: CARBS: PROTEIN: CALORIES:

SNACKS

FAT: CARBS: PROTEIN: CALORIES:

TOP 6 PRIORITIES OF THE DAY

_____

_____

END OF THE DAY TOTAL OVERVIEW

CARBS	FAT	PROTEIN	CALORIES

MY PROGRESS *Tracker*

SLEEP TRACKER:

DATE _____

 RISE: _____

 BEDTIME: _____

 SLEEP (HRS): _____

NOTES FOR THE DAY

_____

_____

_____

IN A STATE OF KETOSIS?

YES   NO   UNSURE

WATER INTAKE TRACKER

EXERCISE / WORKOUT ROUTINE

DAILY ENERGY LEVEL		
HIGH	**MEDIUM**	**LOW**

BREAKFAST

FAT: CARBS: PROTEIN: CALORIES:

LUNCH

FAT: CARBS: PROTEIN: CALORIES:

DINNER

FAT: CARBS: PROTEIN: CALORIES:

SNACKS

FAT: CARBS: PROTEIN: CALORIES:

TOP 6 PRIORITIES OF THE DAY

END OF THE DAY TOTAL OVERVIEW

CARBS	FAT	PROTEIN	CALORIES

MY PROGRESS *Tracker*

SLEEP TRACKER:

DATE _____

 RISE: | BEDTIME: | SLEEP (HRS):

NOTES FOR THE DAY

_____

_____

_____

IN A STATE OF KETOSIS?

YES   NO   UNSURE

WATER INTAKE TRACKER

EXERCISE / WORKOUT ROUTINE

DAILY ENERGY LEVEL		
HIGH	**MEDIUM**	**LOW**

BREAKFAST

FAT: CARBS: PROTEIN: CALORIES:

LUNCH

FAT: CARBS: PROTEIN: CALORIES:

DINNER

FAT: CARBS: PROTEIN: CALORIES:

SNACKS

FAT: CARBS: PROTEIN: CALORIES:

TOP 6 PRIORITIES OF THE DAY

END OF THE DAY TOTAL OVERVIEW

CARBS   FAT   PROTEIN   CALORIES

MY PROGRESS *Tracker*

SLEEP TRACKER:

DATE _____

 RISE: [_____]   🌙 Zᵤᶻ BEDTIME: [_____]   SLEEP (HRS): [_____]

NOTES FOR THE DAY

_____
_____
_____

IN A STATE OF KETOSIS?

YES   NO   UNSURE

WATER INTAKE TRACKER

EXERCISE / WORKOUT ROUTINE

DAILY ENERGY LEVEL		
HIGH	**MEDIUM**	**LOW**

BREAKFAST

FAT: CARBS: PROTEIN: CALORIES:

LUNCH

FAT: CARBS: PROTEIN: CALORIES:

DINNER

FAT: CARBS: PROTEIN: CALORIES:

SNACKS

FAT: CARBS: PROTEIN: CALORIES:

TOP 6 PRIORITIES OF THE DAY

END OF THE DAY TOTAL OVERVIEW

CARBS	FAT	PROTEIN	CALORIES
[ ]	[ ]	[ ]	[ ]

MEAL *Planner*

GROCERY LIST

MON

TUES

WED

THUR

FRI

SAT

SUN

Weekly Meal Planner

Week of: _____

	Breakfast	Lunch	Dinner	Snack	Other
Monday	TOTAL Carbs Fat Protein Cals	TOTAL Carbs Fat Protein Cals	TOTAL Carbs Fat Protein Cals	TOTAL Carbs Fat Protein Cals	TOTAL Carbs Fat Protein Cals
Tuesday	TOTAL Carbs Fat Protein Cals	TOTAL Carbs Fat Protein Cals	TOTAL Carbs Fat Protein Cals	TOTAL Carbs Fat Protein Cals	TOTAL Carbs Fat Protein Cals
Wednesday	TOTAL Carbs Fat Protein Cals	TOTAL Carbs Fat Protein Cals	TOTAL Carbs Fat Protein Cals	TOTAL Carbs Fat Protein Cals	TOTAL Carbs Fat Protein Cals
Thursday	TOTAL Carbs Fat Protein Cals	TOTAL Carbs Fat Protein Cals	TOTAL Carbs Fat Protein Cals	TOTAL Carbs Fat Protein Cals	TOTAL Carbs Fat Protein Cals
Friday	TOTAL Carbs Fat Protein Cals	TOTAL Carbs Fat Protein Cals	TOTAL Carbs Fat Protein Cals	TOTAL Carbs Fat Protein Cals	TOTAL Carbs Fat Protein Cals
Saturday	TOTAL Carbs Fat Protein Cals	TOTAL Carbs Fat Protein Cals	TOTAL Carbs Fat Protein Cals	TOTAL Carbs Fat Protein Cals	TOTAL Carbs Fat Protein Cals
Sunday	TOTAL Carbs Fat Protein Cals	TOTAL Carbs Fat Protein Cals	TOTAL Carbs Fat Protein Cals	TOTAL Carbs Fat Protein Cals	TOTAL Carbs Fat Protein Cals

MY PROGRESS *Tracker*

SLEEP TRACKER:

 RISE: BEDTIME: SLEEP (HRS):

DATE _____

NOTES FOR THE DAY

_____

_____

_____

IN A STATE OF KETOSIS?

YES   NO   UNSURE

WATER INTAKE TRACKER

EXERCISE / WORKOUT ROUTINE

DAILY ENERGY LEVEL		
HIGH	**MEDIUM**	**LOW**

BREAKFAST

FAT: CARBS: PROTEIN: CALORIES:

LUNCH

FAT: CARBS: PROTEIN: CALORIES:

DINNER

FAT: CARBS: PROTEIN: CALORIES:

SNACKS

FAT: CARBS: PROTEIN: CALORIES:

TOP 6 PRIORITIES OF THE DAY

END OF THE DAY TOTAL OVERVIEW

CARBS   FAT   PROTEIN   CALORIES

MY PROGRESS *Tracker*

SLEEP TRACKER:

 DATE _____

 RISE: _____   BEDTIME: _____   SLEEP (HRS): _____

NOTES FOR THE DAY

_____

_____

_____

IN A STATE OF KETOSIS?

YES   NO   UNSURE

WATER INTAKE TRACKER

EXERCISE / WORKOUT ROUTINE

DAILY ENERGY LEVEL		
HIGH	**MEDIUM**	**LOW**

BREAKFAST

FAT: CARBS: PROTEIN: CALORIES:

LUNCH

FAT: CARBS: PROTEIN: CALORIES:

DINNER

FAT: CARBS: PROTEIN: CALORIES:

SNACKS

FAT: CARBS: PROTEIN: CALORIES:

TOP 6 PRIORITIES OF THE DAY

END OF THE DAY TOTAL OVERVIEW

CARBS	FAT	PROTEIN	CALORIES

MY PROGRESS *Tracker*

SLEEP TRACKER:

DATE _____

 RISE: | BEDTIME: | SLEEP (HRS):

NOTES FOR THE DAY

_____

_____

_____

IN A STATE OF KETOSIS?

YES   NO   UNSURE

WATER INTAKE TRACKER

EXERCISE / WORKOUT ROUTINE

DAILY ENERGY LEVEL		
HIGH	**MEDIUM**	**LOW**

BREAKFAST

FAT: CARBS: PROTEIN: CALORIES:

LUNCH

FAT: CARBS: PROTEIN: CALORIES:

DINNER

FAT: CARBS: PROTEIN: CALORIES:

SNACKS

FAT: CARBS: PROTEIN: CALORIES:

TOP 6 PRIORITIES OF THE DAY

END OF THE DAY TOTAL OVERVIEW

CARBS	FAT	PROTEIN	CALORIES

MY PROGRESS *Tracker*

SLEEP TRACKER:

DATE _____

 RISE: _____   BEDTIME: _____   SLEEP (HRS): _____

NOTES FOR THE DAY

_____

_____

_____

IN A STATE OF KETOSIS?

YES   NO   UNSURE

WATER INTAKE TRACKER

EXERCISE / WORKOUT ROUTINE

DAILY ENERGY LEVEL		
HIGH	**MEDIUM**	**LOW**

BREAKFAST

FAT: CARBS: PROTEIN: CALORIES:

LUNCH

FAT: CARBS: PROTEIN: CALORIES:

DINNER

FAT: CARBS: PROTEIN: CALORIES:

SNACKS

FAT: CARBS: PROTEIN: CALORIES:

TOP 6 PRIORITIES OF THE DAY

END OF THE DAY TOTAL OVERVIEW

CARBS	FAT	PROTEIN	CALORIES

MY PROGRESS *Tracker*

SLEEP TRACKER:

DATE _____

 RISE: _____   BEDTIME: _____ SLEEP (HRS): _____

NOTES FOR THE DAY
_____
_____
_____

IN A STATE OF KETOSIS?

YES   NO   UNSURE

WATER INTAKE TRACKER

EXERCISE / WORKOUT ROUTINE

DAILY ENERGY LEVEL		
HIGH	**MEDIUM**	**LOW**

BREAKFAST

FAT: CARBS: PROTEIN: CALORIES:

LUNCH

FAT: CARBS: PROTEIN: CALORIES:

DINNER

FAT: CARBS: PROTEIN: CALORIES:

SNACKS

FAT: CARBS: PROTEIN: CALORIES:

TOP 6 PRIORITIES OF THE DAY

END OF THE DAY TOTAL OVERVIEW

CARBS   FAT   PROTEIN   CALORIES

MY PROGRESS *Tracker*

SLEEP TRACKER:

DATE _____

 RISE: [   ]   BEDTIME: [   ]   SLEEP (HRS): [   ]

NOTES FOR THE DAY

_____

_____

_____

IN A STATE OF KETOSIS?

YES   NO   UNSURE

WATER INTAKE TRACKER

EXERCISE / WORKOUT ROUTINE

DAILY ENERGY LEVEL		
HIGH	**MEDIUM**	**LOW**

BREAKFAST

FAT: CARBS: PROTEIN: CALORIES:

LUNCH

FAT: CARBS: PROTEIN: CALORIES:

DINNER

FAT: CARBS: PROTEIN: CALORIES:

SNACKS

FAT: CARBS: PROTEIN: CALORIES:

TOP 6 PRIORITIES OF THE DAY

END OF THE DAY TOTAL OVERVIEW

CARBS   FAT   PROTEIN   CALORIES

[   ]   [   ]   [   ]   [   ]

MY PROGRESS *Tracker*

SLEEP TRACKER:

DATE _____

 RISE: | BEDTIME: | SLEEP (HRS):

NOTES FOR THE DAY

IN A STATE OF KETOSIS?

YES   NO   UNSURE

WATER INTAKE TRACKER

EXERCISE / WORKOUT ROUTINE

DAILY ENERGY LEVEL		
HIGH	**MEDIUM**	**LOW**

BREAKFAST

FAT: CARBS: PROTEIN: CALORIES:

LUNCH

FAT: CARBS: PROTEIN: CALORIES:

DINNER

FAT: CARBS: PROTEIN: CALORIES:

SNACKS

FAT: CARBS: PROTEIN: CALORIES:

TOP 6 PRIORITIES OF THE DAY

END OF THE DAY TOTAL OVERVIEW

CARBS	FAT	PROTEIN	CALORIES

MEAL *Planner*

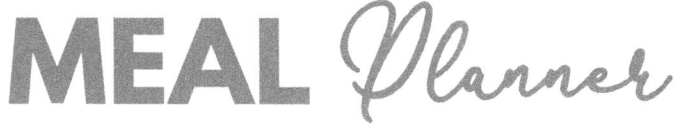

WEEK OF

GROCERY LIST

MON

TUES

WED

THUR

FRI

SAT

SUN

Weekly Meal Planner

Week of: _____

	Breakfast	Lunch	Dinner	Snack	Other
Monday	TOTAL Carbs Fat Protein Cals	TOTAL Carbs Fat Protein Cals	TOTAL Carbs Fat Protein Cals	TOTAL Carbs Fat Protein Cals	TOTAL Carbs Fat Protein Cals
Tuesday	TOTAL Carbs Fat Protein Cals	TOTAL Carbs Fat Protein Cals	TOTAL Carbs Fat Protein Cals	TOTAL Carbs Fat Protein Cals	TOTAL Carbs Fat Protein Cals
Wednesday	TOTAL Carbs Fat Protein Cals	TOTAL Carbs Fat Protein Cals	TOTAL Carbs Fat Protein Cals	TOTAL Carbs Fat Protein Cals	TOTAL Carbs Fat Protein Cals
Thursday	TOTAL Carbs Fat Protein Cals	TOTAL Carbs Fat Protein Cals	TOTAL Carbs Fat Protein Cals	TOTAL Carbs Fat Protein Cals	TOTAL Carbs Fat Protein Cals
Friday	TOTAL Carbs Fat Protein Cals	TOTAL Carbs Fat Protein Cals	TOTAL Carbs Fat Protein Cals	TOTAL Carbs Fat Protein Cals	TOTAL Carbs Fat Protein Cals
Saturday	TOTAL Carbs Fat Protein Cals	TOTAL Carbs Fat Protein Cals	TOTAL Carbs Fat Protein Cals	TOTAL Carbs Fat Protein Cals	TOTAL Carbs Fat Protein Cals
Sunday	TOTAL Carbs Fat Protein Cals	TOTAL Carbs Fat Protein Cals	TOTAL Carbs Fat Protein Cals	TOTAL Carbs Fat Protein Cals	TOTAL Carbs Fat Protein Cals

MY PROGRESS *Tracker*

SLEEP TRACKER: **DATE** _____

 RISE: _____   BEDTIME: _____   SLEEP (HRS): _____

NOTES FOR THE DAY   IN A STATE OF KETOSIS?

_____   YES   NO   UNSURE

_____
                                                WATER INTAKE TRACKER
_____

EXERCISE / WORKOUT ROUTINE

	DAILY ENERGY LEVEL	
HIGH	**MEDIUM**	**LOW**

BREAKFAST

FAT: CARBS: PROTEIN: CALORIES:

LUNCH

FAT: CARBS: PROTEIN: CALORIES:

DINNER

FAT: CARBS: PROTEIN: CALORIES:

SNACKS

FAT: CARBS: PROTEIN: CALORIES:

TOP 6 PRIORITIES OF THE DAY   END OF THE DAY TOTAL OVERVIEW

CARBS   FAT   PROTEIN   CALORIES

MY PROGRESS *Tracker*

SLEEP TRACKER:

DATE _____

 RISE: | BEDTIME: | SLEEP (HRS):

NOTES FOR THE DAY

....

....

....

IN A STATE OF KETOSIS?

YES   NO   UNSURE

WATER INTAKE TRACKER

EXERCISE / WORKOUT ROUTINE

DAILY ENERGY LEVEL		
HIGH	**MEDIUM**	**LOW**

BREAKFAST

FAT: CARBS: PROTEIN: CALORIES:

LUNCH

FAT: CARBS: PROTEIN: CALORIES:

DINNER

FAT: CARBS: PROTEIN: CALORIES:

SNACKS

FAT: CARBS: PROTEIN: CALORIES:

TOP 6 PRIORITIES OF THE DAY

END OF THE DAY TOTAL OVERVIEW

CARBS	FAT	PROTEIN	CALORIES

MY PROGRESS *Tracker*

SLEEP TRACKER:

DATE _____

 RISE: _____   BEDTIME: _____   SLEEP (HRS): _____

NOTES FOR THE DAY

_____

_____

_____

IN A STATE OF KETOSIS?

YES   NO   UNSURE

WATER INTAKE TRACKER

EXERCISE / WORKOUT ROUTINE

DAILY ENERGY LEVEL		
HIGH	**MEDIUM**	**LOW**

BREAKFAST

FAT: CARBS: PROTEIN: CALORIES:

LUNCH

FAT: CARBS: PROTEIN: CALORIES:

DINNER

FAT: CARBS: PROTEIN: CALORIES:

SNACKS

FAT: CARBS: PROTEIN: CALORIES:

TOP 6 PRIORITIES OF THE DAY

END OF THE DAY TOTAL OVERVIEW

CARBS	FAT	PROTEIN	CALORIES

MY PROGRESS *Tracker*

SLEEP TRACKER:

 DATE _____

 RISE: _____   BEDTIME: _____   SLEEP (HRS): _____

NOTES FOR THE DAY

_____

_____

_____

EXERCISE / WORKOUT ROUTINE

IN A STATE OF KETOSIS?

YES   NO   UNSURE

WATER INTAKE TRACKER

DAILY ENERGY LEVEL		
HIGH	**MEDIUM**	**LOW**

BREAKFAST

FAT: CARBS: PROTEIN: CALORIES:

LUNCH

FAT: CARBS: PROTEIN: CALORIES:

DINNER

FAT: CARBS: PROTEIN: CALORIES:

SNACKS

FAT: CARBS: PROTEIN: CALORIES:

TOP 6 PRIORITIES OF THE DAY

END OF THE DAY TOTAL OVERVIEW

CARBS   FAT   PROTEIN   CALORIES

MY PROGRESS *Tracker*

SLEEP TRACKER:

DATE _____

 RISE: _____   BEDTIME: _____   SLEEP (HRS): _____

NOTES FOR THE DAY

_____

_____

_____

IN A STATE OF KETOSIS?

YES   NO   UNSURE

WATER INTAKE TRACKER

EXERCISE / WORKOUT ROUTINE

DAILY ENERGY LEVEL		
HIGH	**MEDIUM**	**LOW**

BREAKFAST

FAT: CARBS: PROTEIN: CALORIES:

LUNCH

FAT: CARBS: PROTEIN: CALORIES:

DINNER

FAT: CARBS: PROTEIN: CALORIES:

SNACKS

FAT: CARBS: PROTEIN: CALORIES:

TOP 6 PRIORITIES OF THE DAY

END OF THE DAY TOTAL OVERVIEW

CARBS	FAT	PROTEIN	CALORIES

MY PROGRESS *Tracker*

SLEEP TRACKER:

DATE _____

☀ RISE: _____   🌙 zzz BEDTIME: _____   💭zzz SLEEP (HRS): _____

NOTES FOR THE DAY

_____
_____
_____

IN A STATE OF KETOSIS?

YES   NO   UNSURE

WATER INTAKE TRACKER

EXERCISE / WORKOUT ROUTINE

DAILY ENERGY LEVEL		
HIGH	**MEDIUM**	**LOW**

BREAKFAST

FAT: CARBS: PROTEIN: CALORIES:

LUNCH

FAT: CARBS: PROTEIN: CALORIES:

DINNER

FAT: CARBS: PROTEIN: CALORIES:

SNACKS

FAT: CARBS: PROTEIN: CALORIES:

TOP 6 PRIORITIES OF THE DAY

_____
_____

END OF THE DAY TOTAL OVERVIEW

CARBS	FAT	PROTEIN	CALORIES

MY PROGRESS *Tracker*

SLEEP TRACKER:

 RISE:

 BEDTIME:

DATE _____

 SLEEP (HRS):

NOTES FOR THE DAY

_____
_____
_____

IN A STATE OF KETOSIS?

YES   NO   UNSURE

WATER INTAKE TRACKER

EXERCISE / WORKOUT ROUTINE

DAILY ENERGY LEVEL		
HIGH	**MEDIUM**	**LOW**

BREAKFAST

FAT: CARBS: PROTEIN: CALORIES:

LUNCH

FAT: CARBS: PROTEIN: CALORIES:

DINNER

FAT: CARBS: PROTEIN: CALORIES:

SNACKS

FAT: CARBS: PROTEIN: CALORIES:

TOP 6 PRIORITIES OF THE DAY

END OF THE DAY TOTAL OVERVIEW

CARBS   FAT   PROTEIN   CALORIES

MEAL *Planner*

GROCERY LIST

MON

TUES

WED

THUR

FRI

SAT

SUN

Weekly Meal Planner

Week of: _____

	Breakfast	Lunch	Dinner	Snack	Other
Monday					
	TOTAL Carbs Fat Protein Cals	TOTAL Carbs Fat Protein Cals	TOTAL Carbs Fat Protein Cals	TOTAL Carbs Fat Protein Cals	TOTAL Carbs Fat Protein Cals
Tuesday					
	TOTAL Carbs Fat Protein Cals	TOTAL Carbs Fat Protein Cals	TOTAL Carbs Fat Protein Cals	TOTAL Carbs Fat Protein Cals	TOTAL Carbs Fat Protein Cals
Wednesday					
	TOTAL Carbs Fat Protein Cals	TOTAL Carbs Fat Protein Cals	TOTAL Carbs Fat Protein Cals	TOTAL Carbs Fat Protein Cals	TOTAL Carbs Fat Protein Cals
Thursday					
	TOTAL Carbs Fat Protein Cals	TOTAL Carbs Fat Protein Cals	TOTAL Carbs Fat Protein Cals	TOTAL Carbs Fat Protein Cals	TOTAL Carbs Fat Protein Cals
Friday					
	TOTAL Carbs Fat Protein Cals	TOTAL Carbs Fat Protein Cals	TOTAL Carbs Fat Protein Cals	TOTAL Carbs Fat Protein Cals	TOTAL Carbs Fat Protein Cals
Saturday					
	TOTAL Carbs Fat Protein Cals	TOTAL Carbs Fat Protein Cals	TOTAL Carbs Fat Protein Cals	TOTAL Carbs Fat Protein Cals	TOTAL Carbs Fat Protein Cals
Sunday					
	TOTAL Carbs Fat Protein Cals	TOTAL Carbs Fat Protein Cals	TOTAL Carbs Fat Protein Cals	TOTAL Carbs Fat Protein Cals	TOTAL Carbs Fat Protein Cals

MY PROGRESS *Tracker*

SLEEP TRACKER:

DATE _____

 RISE: _____

 BEDTIME: _____

 SLEEP (HRS): _____

NOTES FOR THE DAY

_____
_____
_____

IN A STATE OF KETOSIS?

YES   NO   UNSURE

WATER INTAKE TRACKER

EXERCISE / WORKOUT ROUTINE

DAILY ENERGY LEVEL		
HIGH	**MEDIUM**	**LOW**

BREAKFAST

FAT: CARBS: PROTEIN: CALORIES:

LUNCH

FAT: CARBS: PROTEIN: CALORIES:

DINNER

FAT: CARBS: PROTEIN: CALORIES:

SNACKS

FAT: CARBS: PROTEIN: CALORIES:

TOP 6 PRIORITIES OF THE DAY

END OF THE DAY TOTAL OVERVIEW

CARBS   FAT   PROTEIN   CALORIES

MY PROGRESS *Tracker*

SLEEP TRACKER:

DATE _____

 RISE: _____   BEDTIME: _____   SLEEP (HRS): _____

NOTES FOR THE DAY

_____

_____

_____

IN A STATE OF KETOSIS?

YES   NO   UNSURE

WATER INTAKE TRACKER

EXERCISE / WORKOUT ROUTINE

DAILY ENERGY LEVEL		
HIGH	**MEDIUM**	**LOW**

BREAKFAST

FAT: CARBS: PROTEIN: CALORIES:

LUNCH

FAT: CARBS: PROTEIN: CALORIES:

DINNER

FAT: CARBS: PROTEIN: CALORIES:

SNACKS

FAT: CARBS: PROTEIN: CALORIES:

TOP 6 PRIORITIES OF THE DAY

END OF THE DAY TOTAL OVERVIEW

CARBS	FAT	PROTEIN	CALORIES

MY PROGRESS *Tracker*

SLEEP TRACKER:

 RISE:

 BEDTIME:

DATE _____

 SLEEP (HRS):

NOTES FOR THE DAY

_____

_____

_____

IN A STATE OF KETOSIS?

YES   NO   UNSURE

WATER INTAKE TRACKER

EXERCISE / WORKOUT ROUTINE

DAILY ENERGY LEVEL		
HIGH	**MEDIUM**	**LOW**

BREAKFAST

FAT: CARBS: PROTEIN: CALORIES:

LUNCH

FAT: CARBS: PROTEIN: CALORIES:

DINNER

FAT: CARBS: PROTEIN: CALORIES:

SNACKS

FAT: CARBS: PROTEIN: CALORIES:

TOP 6 PRIORITIES OF THE DAY

_____

_____

END OF THE DAY TOTAL OVERVIEW

CARBS	FAT	PROTEIN	CALORIES

MY PROGRESS *Tracker*

SLEEP TRACKER: **DATE** _____

 RISE: _____   BEDTIME: _____   SLEEP (HRS): _____

NOTES FOR THE DAY

_____

_____

_____

IN A STATE OF KETOSIS?

YES   NO   UNSURE

WATER INTAKE TRACKER

EXERCISE / WORKOUT ROUTINE

DAILY ENERGY LEVEL		
HIGH	**MEDIUM**	**LOW**

BREAKFAST

FAT: CARBS: PROTEIN: CALORIES:

LUNCH

FAT: CARBS: PROTEIN: CALORIES:

DINNER

FAT: CARBS: PROTEIN: CALORIES:

SNACKS

FAT: CARBS: PROTEIN: CALORIES:

TOP 6 PRIORITIES OF THE DAY

END OF THE DAY TOTAL OVERVIEW

CARBS   FAT   PROTEIN   CALORIES

MY PROGRESS *Tracker*

SLEEP TRACKER:

DATE _____

☼ RISE: _____   🌙 zᵤz BEDTIME: _____   ☁zᶻz SLEEP (HRS): _____

NOTES FOR THE DAY

_____

_____

_____

IN A STATE OF KETOSIS?

YES   NO   UNSURE

WATER INTAKE TRACKER

EXERCISE / WORKOUT ROUTINE

DAILY ENERGY LEVEL		
HIGH	**MEDIUM**	**LOW**

BREAKFAST

FAT: CARBS: PROTEIN: CALORIES:

LUNCH

FAT: CARBS: PROTEIN: CALORIES:

DINNER

FAT: CARBS: PROTEIN: CALORIES:

SNACKS

FAT: CARBS: PROTEIN: CALORIES:

TOP 6 PRIORITIES OF THE DAY

END OF THE DAY TOTAL OVERVIEW

CARBS	FAT	PROTEIN	CALORIES
☐	☐	☐	☐

MY PROGRESS *Tracker*

SLEEP TRACKER:

DATE _____

 RISE: [　　　　]　　 BEDTIME: [　　　　]　　 SLEEP (HRS): [　　　　]

NOTES FOR THE DAY

_____

_____

IN A STATE OF KETOSIS?

YES　　　NO　　　UNSURE

WATER INTAKE TRACKER

EXERCISE / WORKOUT ROUTINE

DAILY ENERGY LEVEL		
HIGH	**MEDIUM**	**LOW**

BREAKFAST

FAT:　　CARBS:　　PROTEIN:　　CALORIES:

LUNCH

FAT:　　CARBS:　　PROTEIN:　　CALORIES:

DINNER

FAT:　　CARBS:　　PROTEIN:　　CALORIES:

SNACKS

FAT:　　CARBS:　　PROTEIN:　　CALORIES:

TOP 6 PRIORITIES OF THE DAY

END OF THE DAY TOTAL OVERVIEW

CARBS	FAT	PROTEIN	CALORIES

MY PROGRESS *Tracker*

SLEEP TRACKER:

 RISE: BEDTIME: SLEEP (HRS):

DATE _____

NOTES FOR THE DAY

_____
_____
_____

IN A STATE OF KETOSIS?

YES   NO   UNSURE

WATER INTAKE TRACKER

EXERCISE / WORKOUT ROUTINE

DAILY ENERGY LEVEL		
HIGH	**MEDIUM**	**LOW**

BREAKFAST

FAT: CARBS: PROTEIN: CALORIES:

LUNCH

FAT: CARBS: PROTEIN: CALORIES:

DINNER

FAT: CARBS: PROTEIN: CALORIES:

SNACKS

FAT: CARBS: PROTEIN: CALORIES:

TOP 6 PRIORITIES OF THE DAY

END OF THE DAY TOTAL OVERVIEW

CARBS	FAT	PROTEIN	CALORIES

MEAL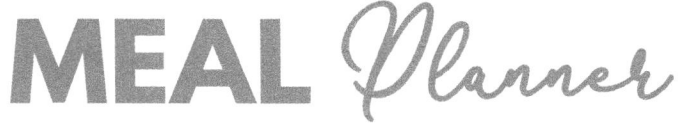

WEEK OF

GROCERY LIST

MON

TUES

WED

THUR

FRI

SAT

SUN

Weekly Meal Planner

Week of: _____

	Breakfast	Lunch	Dinner	Snack	Other
Monday	TOTAL Carbs Fat Protein Cals	TOTAL Carbs Fat Protein Cals	TOTAL Carbs Fat Protein Cals	TOTAL Carbs Fat Protein Cals	TOTAL Carbs Fat Protein Cals
Tuesday	TOTAL Carbs Fat Protein Cals	TOTAL Carbs Fat Protein Cals	TOTAL Carbs Fat Protein Cals	TOTAL Carbs Fat Protein Cals	TOTAL Carbs Fat Protein Cals
Wednesday	TOTAL Carbs Fat Protein Cals	TOTAL Carbs Fat Protein Cals	TOTAL Carbs Fat Protein Cals	TOTAL Carbs Fat Protein Cals	TOTAL Carbs Fat Protein Cals
Thursday	TOTAL Carbs Fat Protein Cals	TOTAL Carbs Fat Protein Cals	TOTAL Carbs Fat Protein Cals	TOTAL Carbs Fat Protein Cals	TOTAL Carbs Fat Protein Cals
Friday	TOTAL Carbs Fat Protein Cals	TOTAL Carbs Fat Protein Cals	TOTAL Carbs Fat Protein Cals	TOTAL Carbs Fat Protein Cals	TOTAL Carbs Fat Protein Cals
Saturday	TOTAL Carbs Fat Protein Cals	TOTAL Carbs Fat Protein Cals	TOTAL Carbs Fat Protein Cals	TOTAL Carbs Fat Protein Cals	TOTAL Carbs Fat Protein Cals
Sunday	TOTAL Carbs Fat Protein Cals	TOTAL Carbs Fat Protein Cals	TOTAL Carbs Fat Protein Cals	TOTAL Carbs Fat Protein Cals	TOTAL Carbs Fat Protein Cals

MY PROGRESS *Tracker*

SLEEP TRACKER:

DATE _____

 RISE: _____   BEDTIME: _____   SLEEP (HRS): _____

NOTES FOR THE DAY

_____

_____

_____

IN A STATE OF KETOSIS?

YES   NO   UNSURE

WATER INTAKE TRACKER

EXERCISE / WORKOUT ROUTINE

DAILY ENERGY LEVEL		
HIGH	**MEDIUM**	**LOW**

BREAKFAST

FAT: CARBS: PROTEIN: CALORIES:

LUNCH

FAT: CARBS: PROTEIN: CALORIES:

DINNER

FAT: CARBS: PROTEIN: CALORIES:

SNACKS

FAT: CARBS: PROTEIN: CALORIES:

TOP 6 PRIORITIES OF THE DAY

END OF THE DAY TOTAL OVERVIEW

CARBS	FAT	PROTEIN	CALORIES

MY PROGRESS *Tracker*

SLEEP TRACKER:

DATE _____

 RISE: _____   BEDTIME: _____   SLEEP (HRS): _____

NOTES FOR THE DAY

_____
_____
_____

IN A STATE OF KETOSIS?

YES   NO   UNSURE

WATER INTAKE TRACKER

EXERCISE / WORKOUT ROUTINE

DAILY ENERGY LEVEL		
HIGH	**MEDIUM**	**LOW**

BREAKFAST

FAT: CARBS: PROTEIN: CALORIES:

LUNCH

FAT: CARBS: PROTEIN: CALORIES:

DINNER

FAT: CARBS: PROTEIN: CALORIES:

SNACKS

FAT: CARBS: PROTEIN: CALORIES:

TOP 6 PRIORITIES OF THE DAY

END OF THE DAY TOTAL OVERVIEW

CARBS   FAT   PROTEIN   CALORIES

MY PROGRESS *Tracker*

SLEEP TRACKER:

 RISE: _____

 BEDTIME: _____

DATE _____

 SLEEP (HRS): _____

NOTES FOR THE DAY

_____

_____

_____

IN A STATE OF KETOSIS?

YES   NO   UNSURE

WATER INTAKE TRACKER

EXERCISE / WORKOUT ROUTINE

DAILY ENERGY LEVEL		
HIGH	**MEDIUM**	**LOW**

BREAKFAST

FAT: CARBS: PROTEIN: CALORIES:

LUNCH

FAT: CARBS: PROTEIN: CALORIES:

DINNER

FAT: CARBS: PROTEIN: CALORIES:

SNACKS

FAT: CARBS: PROTEIN: CALORIES:

TOP 6 PRIORITIES OF THE DAY

END OF THE DAY TOTAL OVERVIEW

CARBS	FAT	PROTEIN	CALORIES

MY PROGRESS *Tracker*

SLEEP TRACKER:

 RISE: _____

BEDTIME: _____

 SLEEP (HRS): _____

NOTES FOR THE DAY

_____

_____

IN A STATE OF KETOSIS?

YES   NO   UNSURE

WATER INTAKE TRACKER

EXERCISE / WORKOUT ROUTINE

DAILY ENERGY LEVEL		
HIGH	**MEDIUM**	**LOW**

BREAKFAST

FAT: CARBS: PROTEIN: CALORIES:

LUNCH

FAT: CARBS: PROTEIN: CALORIES:

DINNER

FAT: CARBS: PROTEIN: CALORIES:

SNACKS

FAT: CARBS: PROTEIN: CALORIES:

TOP 6 PRIORITIES OF THE DAY

END OF THE DAY TOTAL OVERVIEW

CARBS	FAT	PROTEIN	CALORIES
☐	☐	☐	☐

MY PROGRESS *Tracker*

SLEEP TRACKER:

DATE _____

 RISE: | BEDTIME: | SLEEP (HRS):

NOTES FOR THE DAY

_____
_____
_____

IN A STATE OF KETOSIS?

YES   NO   UNSURE

WATER INTAKE TRACKER

EXERCISE / WORKOUT ROUTINE

DAILY ENERGY LEVEL		
HIGH	**MEDIUM**	**LOW**

BREAKFAST

FAT: CARBS: PROTEIN: CALORIES:

LUNCH

FAT: CARBS: PROTEIN: CALORIES:

DINNER

FAT: CARBS: PROTEIN: CALORIES:

SNACKS

FAT: CARBS: PROTEIN: CALORIES:

TOP 6 PRIORITIES OF THE DAY

END OF THE DAY TOTAL OVERVIEW

CARBS	FAT	PROTEIN	CALORIES

MY PROGRESS *Tracker*

SLEEP TRACKER:

DATE _____

 RISE: [_____]   BEDTIME: [_____]   SLEEP (HRS): [_____]

NOTES FOR THE DAY

_____

_____

_____

IN A STATE OF KETOSIS?

YES   NO   UNSURE

WATER INTAKE TRACKER

EXERCISE / WORKOUT ROUTINE

DAILY ENERGY LEVEL		
HIGH	**MEDIUM**	**LOW**

BREAKFAST

FAT: CARBS: PROTEIN: CALORIES:

LUNCH

FAT: CARBS: PROTEIN: CALORIES:

DINNER

FAT: CARBS: PROTEIN: CALORIES:

SNACKS

FAT: CARBS: PROTEIN: CALORIES:

TOP 6 PRIORITIES OF THE DAY

END OF THE DAY TOTAL OVERVIEW

CARBS	FAT	PROTEIN	CALORIES
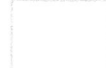			

MY PROGRESS *Tracker*

SLEEP TRACKER:

DATE _____

☀ RISE: _____ 🌙 ᶻᶻᶻ BEDTIME: _____ 💭ᶻᶻᶻ SLEEP (HRS): _____

NOTES FOR THE DAY

_____

_____

_____

IN A STATE OF KETOSIS?

YES   NO   UNSURE

WATER INTAKE TRACKER

EXERCISE / WORKOUT ROUTINE

DAILY ENERGY LEVEL		
HIGH	**MEDIUM**	**LOW**

BREAKFAST

FAT: CARBS: PROTEIN: CALORIES:

LUNCH

FAT: CARBS: PROTEIN: CALORIES:

DINNER

FAT: CARBS: PROTEIN: CALORIES:

SNACKS

FAT: CARBS: PROTEIN: CALORIES:

TOP 6 PRIORITIES OF THE DAY

END OF THE DAY TOTAL OVERVIEW

CARBS   FAT   PROTEIN   CALORIES

MEAL *Planner*

WEEK OF

GROCERY LIST

MON

TUES

WED

THUR

FRI

SAT

SUN

Weekly Meal Planner

Week of: _____

	Breakfast	Lunch	Dinner	Snack	Other
Monday	TOTAL Carbs Fat Protein Cals	TOTAL Carbs Fat Protein Cals	TOTAL Carbs Fat Protein Cals	TOTAL Carbs Fat Protein Cals	TOTAL Carbs Fat Protein Cals
Tuesday	TOTAL Carbs Fat Protein Cals	TOTAL Carbs Fat Protein Cals	TOTAL Carbs Fat Protein Cals	TOTAL Carbs Fat Protein Cals	TOTAL Carbs Fat Protein Cals
Wednesday	TOTAL Carbs Fat Protein Cals	TOTAL Carbs Fat Protein Cals	TOTAL Carbs Fat Protein Cals	TOTAL Carbs Fat Protein Cals	TOTAL Carbs Fat Protein Cals
Thursday	TOTAL Carbs Fat Protein Cals	TOTAL Carbs Fat Protein Cals	TOTAL Carbs Fat Protein Cals	TOTAL Carbs Fat Protein Cals	TOTAL Carbs Fat Protein Cals
Friday	TOTAL Carbs Fat Protein Cals	TOTAL Carbs Fat Protein Cals	TOTAL Carbs Fat Protein Cals	TOTAL Carbs Fat Protein Cals	TOTAL Carbs Fat Protein Cals
Saturday	TOTAL Carbs Fat Protein Cals	TOTAL Carbs Fat Protein Cals	TOTAL Carbs Fat Protein Cals	TOTAL Carbs Fat Protein Cals	TOTAL Carbs Fat Protein Cals
Sunday	TOTAL Carbs Fat Protein Cals	TOTAL Carbs Fat Protein Cals	TOTAL Carbs Fat Protein Cals	TOTAL Carbs Fat Protein Cals	TOTAL Carbs Fat Protein Cals

MY PROGRESS *Tracker*

SLEEP TRACKER:

DATE _____

 RISE: _____   BEDTIME: _____   SLEEP (HRS): _____

NOTES FOR THE DAY

_____

_____

_____

IN A STATE OF KETOSIS?

YES   NO   UNSURE

WATER INTAKE TRACKER

EXERCISE / WORKOUT ROUTINE

DAILY ENERGY LEVEL		
HIGH	**MEDIUM**	**LOW**

BREAKFAST

FAT: CARBS: PROTEIN: CALORIES:

LUNCH

FAT: CARBS: PROTEIN: CALORIES:

DINNER

FAT: CARBS: PROTEIN: CALORIES:

SNACKS

FAT: CARBS: PROTEIN: CALORIES:

TOP 6 PRIORITIES OF THE DAY

END OF THE DAY TOTAL OVERVIEW

CARBS	FAT	PROTEIN	CALORIES

MY PROGRESS *Tracker*

SLEEP TRACKER:

DATE _____

 RISE: _____   BEDTIME: _____   SLEEP (HRS): _____

NOTES FOR THE DAY

_____

_____

_____

IN A STATE OF KETOSIS?

YES   NO   UNSURE

WATER INTAKE TRACKER

EXERCISE / WORKOUT ROUTINE

DAILY ENERGY LEVEL		
HIGH	**MEDIUM**	**LOW**

BREAKFAST

FAT: CARBS: PROTEIN: CALORIES:

LUNCH

FAT: CARBS: PROTEIN: CALORIES:

DINNER

FAT: CARBS: PROTEIN: CALORIES:

SNACKS

FAT: CARBS: PROTEIN: CALORIES:

TOP 6 PRIORITIES OF THE DAY

END OF THE DAY TOTAL OVERVIEW

CARBS	FAT	PROTEIN	CALORIES

MY PROGRESS *Tracker*

SLEEP TRACKER:

DATE _____

☼ RISE: _____ 🌙ᶻᶻᶻ BEDTIME: _____ 💭ᶻᶻᶻ SLEEP (HRS): _____

NOTES FOR THE DAY

_____

_____

IN A STATE OF KETOSIS?

YES   NO   UNSURE

WATER INTAKE TRACKER

EXERCISE / WORKOUT ROUTINE

DAILY ENERGY LEVEL		
HIGH	**MEDIUM**	**LOW**

BREAKFAST

FAT: CARBS: PROTEIN: CALORIES:

LUNCH

FAT: CARBS: PROTEIN: CALORIES:

DINNER

FAT: CARBS: PROTEIN: CALORIES:

SNACKS

FAT: CARBS: PROTEIN: CALORIES:

TOP 6 PRIORITIES OF THE DAY

END OF THE DAY TOTAL OVERVIEW

CARBS	FAT	PROTEIN	CALORIES
☐	☐	☐	☐

MY PROGRESS *Tracker*

SLEEP TRACKER:

DATE _____

 RISE: _____   BEDTIME: _____   SLEEP (HRS): _____

NOTES FOR THE DAY

_____

_____

_____

IN A STATE OF KETOSIS?

YES   NO   UNSURE

WATER INTAKE TRACKER

EXERCISE / WORKOUT ROUTINE

DAILY ENERGY LEVEL		
HIGH	**MEDIUM**	**LOW**

BREAKFAST

FAT: CARBS: PROTEIN: CALORIES:

LUNCH

FAT: CARBS: PROTEIN: CALORIES:

DINNER

FAT: CARBS: PROTEIN: CALORIES:

SNACKS

FAT: CARBS: PROTEIN: CALORIES:

TOP 6 PRIORITIES OF THE DAY

_____

_____

END OF THE DAY TOTAL OVERVIEW

CARBS	FAT	PROTEIN	CALORIES

MY PROGRESS *Tracker*

SLEEP TRACKER:

 RISE: _____

 BEDTIME: _____

 SLEEP (HRS): _____

NOTES FOR THE DAY

_____

_____

_____

IN A STATE OF KETOSIS?

YES   NO   UNSURE

WATER INTAKE TRACKER

EXERCISE / WORKOUT ROUTINE

DAILY ENERGY LEVEL		
HIGH	**MEDIUM**	**LOW**

BREAKFAST

FAT: CARBS: PROTEIN: CALORIES:

LUNCH

FAT: CARBS: PROTEIN: CALORIES:

DINNER

FAT: CARBS: PROTEIN: CALORIES:

SNACKS

FAT: CARBS: PROTEIN: CALORIES:

TOP 6 PRIORITIES OF THE DAY

_____

_____

_____

END OF THE DAY TOTAL OVERVIEW

CARBS	FAT	PROTEIN	CALORIES

MY PROGRESS *Tracker*

SLEEP TRACKER:

DATE _____

 RISE: | BEDTIME: | SLEEP (HRS):

NOTES FOR THE DAY

_____
_____
_____

EXERCISE / WORKOUT ROUTINE

IN A STATE OF KETOSIS?

YES   NO   UNSURE

WATER INTAKE TRACKER

DAILY ENERGY LEVEL		
HIGH	**MEDIUM**	**LOW**

BREAKFAST

FAT: CARBS: PROTEIN: CALORIES:

LUNCH

FAT: CARBS: PROTEIN: CALORIES:

DINNER

FAT: CARBS: PROTEIN: CALORIES:

SNACKS

FAT: CARBS: PROTEIN: CALORIES:

TOP 6 PRIORITIES OF THE DAY

END OF THE DAY TOTAL OVERVIEW

CARBS	FAT	PROTEIN	CALORIES

MY PROGRESS *Tracker*

SLEEP TRACKER:

 RISE: BEDTIME: SLEEP (HRS):

DATE _____

NOTES FOR THE DAY

_____

_____

_____

IN A STATE OF KETOSIS?

YES   NO   UNSURE

WATER INTAKE TRACKER

EXERCISE / WORKOUT ROUTINE

DAILY ENERGY LEVEL		
HIGH	**MEDIUM**	**LOW**

BREAKFAST

FAT: CARBS: PROTEIN: CALORIES:

LUNCH

FAT: CARBS: PROTEIN: CALORIES:

DINNER

FAT: CARBS: PROTEIN: CALORIES:

SNACKS

FAT: CARBS: PROTEIN: CALORIES:

TOP 6 PRIORITIES OF THE DAY

_____

_____

END OF THE DAY TOTAL OVERVIEW

CARBS	FAT	PROTEIN	CALORIES

MEAL *Planner*

GROCERY LIST

MON

TUES

WED

THUR

FRI

SAT

SUN

Weekly Meal Planner

Week of: _____

	Breakfast	Lunch	Dinner	Snack	Other
Monday	TOTAL Carbs Fat Protein Cals	TOTAL Carbs Fat Protein Cals	TOTAL Carbs Fat Protein Cals	TOTAL Carbs Fat Protein Cals	TOTAL Carbs Fat Protein Cals
Tuesday	TOTAL Carbs Fat Protein Cals	TOTAL Carbs Fat Protein Cals	TOTAL Carbs Fat Protein Cals	TOTAL Carbs Fat Protein Cals	TOTAL Carbs Fat Protein Cals
Wednesday	TOTAL Carbs Fat Protein Cals	TOTAL Carbs Fat Protein Cals	TOTAL Carbs Fat Protein Cals	TOTAL Carbs Fat Protein Cals	TOTAL Carbs Fat Protein Cals
Thursday	TOTAL Carbs Fat Protein Cals	TOTAL Carbs Fat Protein Cals	TOTAL Carbs Fat Protein Cals	TOTAL Carbs Fat Protein Cals	TOTAL Carbs Fat Protein Cals
Friday	TOTAL Carbs Fat Protein Cals	TOTAL Carbs Fat Protein Cals	TOTAL Carbs Fat Protein Cals	TOTAL Carbs Fat Protein Cals	TOTAL Carbs Fat Protein Cals
Saturday	TOTAL Carbs Fat Protein Cals	TOTAL Carbs Fat Protein Cals	TOTAL Carbs Fat Protein Cals	TOTAL Carbs Fat Protein Cals	TOTAL Carbs Fat Protein Cals
Sunday	TOTAL Carbs Fat Protein Cals	TOTAL Carbs Fat Protein Cals	TOTAL Carbs Fat Protein Cals	TOTAL Carbs Fat Protein Cals	TOTAL Carbs Fat Protein Cals

MY PROGRESS *Tracker*

SLEEP TRACKER:

DATE _____

 RISE: _____

 BEDTIME: _____

 SLEEP (HRS): _____

NOTES FOR THE DAY

_____

_____

_____

IN A STATE OF KETOSIS?

YES   NO   UNSURE

WATER INTAKE TRACKER

EXERCISE / WORKOUT ROUTINE

DAILY ENERGY LEVEL		
HIGH	**MEDIUM**	**LOW**

BREAKFAST

FAT: CARBS: PROTEIN: CALORIES:

LUNCH

FAT: CARBS: PROTEIN: CALORIES:

DINNER

FAT: CARBS: PROTEIN: CALORIES:

SNACKS

FAT: CARBS: PROTEIN: CALORIES:

TOP 6 PRIORITIES OF THE DAY

END OF THE DAY TOTAL OVERVIEW

CARBS	FAT	PROTEIN	CALORIES

MY PROGRESS *Tracker*

SLEEP TRACKER:

☼ RISE: _____   🌙 zzz BEDTIME: _____   💭 zzz SLEEP (HRS): _____

NOTES FOR THE DAY

_____

_____

_____

IN A STATE OF KETOSIS?

YES   NO   UNSURE

WATER INTAKE TRACKER

EXERCISE / WORKOUT ROUTINE

DAILY ENERGY LEVEL		
HIGH	**MEDIUM**	**LOW**

BREAKFAST

FAT: CARBS: PROTEIN: CALORIES:

LUNCH

FAT: CARBS: PROTEIN: CALORIES:

DINNER

FAT: CARBS: PROTEIN: CALORIES:

SNACKS

FAT: CARBS: PROTEIN: CALORIES:

TOP 6 PRIORITIES OF THE DAY

_____

_____

END OF THE DAY TOTAL OVERVIEW

CARBS	FAT	PROTEIN	CALORIES

MY PROGRESS *Tracker*

SLEEP TRACKER:

DATE _____

 RISE: [   ]   BEDTIME: [   ]   SLEEP (HRS): [   ]

NOTES FOR THE DAY

_____

_____

IN A STATE OF KETOSIS?

YES   NO   UNSURE

WATER INTAKE TRACKER

EXERCISE / WORKOUT ROUTINE

DAILY ENERGY LEVEL		
HIGH	**MEDIUM**	**LOW**

BREAKFAST

FAT: CARBS: PROTEIN: CALORIES:

LUNCH

FAT: CARBS: PROTEIN: CALORIES:

DINNER

FAT: CARBS: PROTEIN: CALORIES:

SNACKS

FAT: CARBS: PROTEIN: CALORIES:

TOP 6 PRIORITIES OF THE DAY

END OF THE DAY TOTAL OVERVIEW

CARBS	FAT	PROTEIN	CALORIES
[ ]	[ ]	[ ]	[ ]

MY PROGRESS *Tracker*

SLEEP TRACKER:

 RISE: BEDTIME: SLEEP (HRS):

DATE _____

NOTES FOR THE DAY

_____

_____

_____

IN A STATE OF KETOSIS?

YES   NO   UNSURE

WATER INTAKE TRACKER

EXERCISE / WORKOUT ROUTINE

DAILY ENERGY LEVEL		
HIGH	**MEDIUM**	**LOW**

BREAKFAST

FAT: CARBS: PROTEIN: CALORIES:

LUNCH

FAT: CARBS: PROTEIN: CALORIES:

DINNER

FAT: CARBS: PROTEIN: CALORIES:

SNACKS

FAT: CARBS: PROTEIN: CALORIES:

TOP 6 PRIORITIES OF THE DAY

_____

_____

END OF THE DAY TOTAL OVERVIEW

CARBS	FAT	PROTEIN	CALORIES

MY PROGRESS *Tracker*

SLEEP TRACKER:

DATE _____

 RISE: BEDTIME: SLEEP (HRS):

NOTES FOR THE DAY

_____

_____

_____

IN A STATE OF KETOSIS?

YES   NO   UNSURE

WATER INTAKE TRACKER

EXERCISE / WORKOUT ROUTINE

DAILY ENERGY LEVEL		
HIGH	**MEDIUM**	**LOW**

BREAKFAST

FAT: CARBS: PROTEIN: CALORIES:

LUNCH

FAT: CARBS: PROTEIN: CALORIES:

DINNER

FAT: CARBS: PROTEIN: CALORIES:

SNACKS

FAT: CARBS: PROTEIN: CALORIES:

TOP 6 PRIORITIES OF THE DAY

END OF THE DAY TOTAL OVERVIEW

CARBS	FAT	PROTEIN	CALORIES

MY PROGRESS *Tracker*

SLEEP TRACKER:

DATE _____

 RISE: _____   BEDTIME: _____   SLEEP (HRS): _____

NOTES FOR THE DAY

_____
_____
_____

IN A STATE OF KETOSIS?

YES   NO   UNSURE

WATER INTAKE TRACKER

EXERCISE / WORKOUT ROUTINE

DAILY ENERGY LEVEL		
HIGH	**MEDIUM**	**LOW**

BREAKFAST

FAT: CARBS: PROTEIN: CALORIES:

LUNCH

FAT: CARBS: PROTEIN: CALORIES:

DINNER

FAT: CARBS: PROTEIN: CALORIES:

SNACKS

FAT: CARBS: PROTEIN: CALORIES:

TOP 6 PRIORITIES OF THE DAY

END OF THE DAY TOTAL OVERVIEW

CARBS	FAT	PROTEIN	CALORIES

MY PROGRESS *Tracker*

SLEEP TRACKER:

DATE _____

 RISE: _____   BEDTIME: _____   SLEEP (HRS): _____

NOTES FOR THE DAY

_____
_____
_____

IN A STATE OF KETOSIS?

YES   NO   UNSURE

WATER INTAKE TRACKER

EXERCISE / WORKOUT ROUTINE

DAILY ENERGY LEVEL		
HIGH	**MEDIUM**	**LOW**

BREAKFAST

FAT: CARBS: PROTEIN: CALORIES:

LUNCH

FAT: CARBS: PROTEIN: CALORIES:

DINNER

FAT: CARBS: PROTEIN: CALORIES:

SNACKS

FAT: CARBS: PROTEIN: CALORIES:

TOP 6 PRIORITIES OF THE DAY

END OF THE DAY TOTAL OVERVIEW

CARBS	FAT	PROTEIN	CALORIES

MEAL Planner

GROCERY LIST

MON

TUES

WED

THUR

FRI

SAT

SUN

Weekly Meal Planner

Week of: _____

	Breakfast	Lunch	Dinner	Snack	Other
Monday	TOTAL — Carbs Fat Protein Cals	TOTAL — Carbs Fat Protein Cals	TOTAL — Carbs Fat Protein Cals	TOTAL — Carbs Fat Protein Cals	TOTAL — Carbs Fat Protein Cals
Tuesday	TOTAL — Carbs Fat Protein Cals	TOTAL — Carbs Fat Protein Cals	TOTAL — Carbs Fat Protein Cals	TOTAL — Carbs Fat Protein Cals	TOTAL — Carbs Fat Protein Cals
Wednesday	TOTAL — Carbs Fat Protein Cals	TOTAL — Carbs Fat Protein Cals	TOTAL — Carbs Fat Protein Cals	TOTAL — Carbs Fat Protein Cals	TOTAL — Carbs Fat Protein Cals
Thursday	TOTAL — Carbs Fat Protein Cals	TOTAL — Carbs Fat Protein Cals	TOTAL — Carbs Fat Protein Cals	TOTAL — Carbs Fat Protein Cals	TOTAL — Carbs Fat Protein Cals
Friday	TOTAL — Carbs Fat Protein Cals	TOTAL — Carbs Fat Protein Cals	TOTAL — Carbs Fat Protein Cals	TOTAL — Carbs Fat Protein Cals	TOTAL — Carbs Fat Protein Cals
Saturday	TOTAL — Carbs Fat Protein Cals	TOTAL — Carbs Fat Protein Cals	TOTAL — Carbs Fat Protein Cals	TOTAL — Carbs Fat Protein Cals	TOTAL — Carbs Fat Protein Cals
Sunday	TOTAL — Carbs Fat Protein Cals	TOTAL — Carbs Fat Protein Cals	TOTAL — Carbs Fat Protein Cals	TOTAL — Carbs Fat Protein Cals	TOTAL — Carbs Fat Protein Cals

MY PROGRESS *Tracker*

SLEEP TRACKER:

DATE _____

☀ RISE: _____   🌙 zzz BEDTIME: _____   💭 zzz SLEEP (HRS): _____

NOTES FOR THE DAY

_____
_____
_____

IN A STATE OF KETOSIS?

YES   NO   UNSURE

WATER INTAKE TRACKER

EXERCISE / WORKOUT ROUTINE

DAILY ENERGY LEVEL		
HIGH	**MEDIUM**	**LOW**

BREAKFAST

FAT: CARBS: PROTEIN: CALORIES:

LUNCH

FAT: CARBS: PROTEIN: CALORIES:

DINNER

FAT: CARBS: PROTEIN: CALORIES:

SNACKS

FAT: CARBS: PROTEIN: CALORIES:

TOP 6 PRIORITIES OF THE DAY

END OF THE DAY TOTAL OVERVIEW

CARBS	FAT	PROTEIN	CALORIES

MY PROGRESS *Tracker*

SLEEP TRACKER:

DATE _____

 RISE: _____   BEDTIME: _____   SLEEP (HRS): _____

NOTES FOR THE DAY

_____

_____

_____

IN A STATE OF KETOSIS?

YES   NO   UNSURE

WATER INTAKE TRACKER

EXERCISE / WORKOUT ROUTINE

DAILY ENERGY LEVEL		
HIGH	**MEDIUM**	**LOW**

BREAKFAST

FAT: CARBS: PROTEIN: CALORIES:

LUNCH

FAT: CARBS: PROTEIN: CALORIES:

DINNER

FAT: CARBS: PROTEIN: CALORIES:

SNACKS

FAT: CARBS: PROTEIN: CALORIES:

TOP 6 PRIORITIES OF THE DAY

END OF THE DAY TOTAL OVERVIEW

CARBS	FAT	PROTEIN	CALORIES

MY PROGRESS *Tracker*

SLEEP TRACKER:

 RISE:

 BEDTIME:

DATE _____

 SLEEP (HRS):

NOTES FOR THE DAY

_____
_____
_____

IN A STATE OF KETOSIS?

YES   NO   UNSURE

WATER INTAKE TRACKER

EXERCISE / WORKOUT ROUTINE

DAILY ENERGY LEVEL		
HIGH	**MEDIUM**	**LOW**

BREAKFAST

FAT: CARBS: PROTEIN: CALORIES:

LUNCH

FAT: CARBS: PROTEIN: CALORIES:

DINNER

FAT: CARBS: PROTEIN: CALORIES:

SNACKS

FAT: CARBS: PROTEIN: CALORIES:

TOP 6 PRIORITIES OF THE DAY

_____
_____

END OF THE DAY TOTAL OVERVIEW

CARBS   FAT   PROTEIN   CALORIES

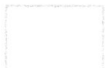 

MY PROGRESS *Tracker*

SLEEP TRACKER:

DATE _____

 RISE: _____   BEDTIME: _____   SLEEP (HRS): _____

NOTES FOR THE DAY

_____

_____

_____

IN A STATE OF KETOSIS?

YES   NO   UNSURE

WATER INTAKE TRACKER

EXERCISE / WORKOUT ROUTINE

DAILY ENERGY LEVEL		
HIGH	**MEDIUM**	**LOW**

BREAKFAST

FAT: CARBS: PROTEIN: CALORIES:

LUNCH

FAT: CARBS: PROTEIN: CALORIES:

DINNER

FAT: CARBS: PROTEIN: CALORIES:

SNACKS

FAT: CARBS: PROTEIN: CALORIES:

TOP 6 PRIORITIES OF THE DAY

END OF THE DAY TOTAL OVERVIEW

CARBS   FAT   PROTEIN   CALORIES

MY PROGRESS *Tracker*

SLEEP TRACKER:

DATE _____

☀ RISE: | 🌙 zᶻᶻ BEDTIME: | 💭 zᶻᶻ SLEEP (HRS):

NOTES FOR THE DAY

_____

_____

_____

IN A STATE OF KETOSIS?

YES   NO   UNSURE

WATER INTAKE TRACKER

EXERCISE / WORKOUT ROUTINE

DAILY ENERGY LEVEL		
HIGH	**MEDIUM**	**LOW**

BREAKFAST

FAT: CARBS: PROTEIN: CALORIES:

LUNCH

FAT: CARBS: PROTEIN: CALORIES:

DINNER

FAT: CARBS: PROTEIN: CALORIES:

SNACKS

FAT: CARBS: PROTEIN: CALORIES:

TOP 6 PRIORITIES OF THE DAY

END OF THE DAY TOTAL OVERVIEW

CARBS	FAT	PROTEIN	CALORIES

MY PROGRESS *Tracker*

SLEEP TRACKER:

 RISE: BEDTIME: SLEEP (HRS):

DATE _____

NOTES FOR THE DAY

_____

_____

IN A STATE OF KETOSIS?

YES   NO   UNSURE

WATER INTAKE TRACKER

EXERCISE / WORKOUT ROUTINE

DAILY ENERGY LEVEL

HIGH	MEDIUM	LOW

BREAKFAST

FAT: CARBS: PROTEIN: CALORIES:

LUNCH

FAT: CARBS: PROTEIN: CALORIES:

DINNER

FAT: CARBS: PROTEIN: CALORIES:

SNACKS

FAT: CARBS: PROTEIN: CALORIES:

TOP 6 PRIORITIES OF THE DAY

END OF THE DAY TOTAL OVERVIEW

CARBS	FAT	PROTEIN	CALORIES

MY PROGRESS *Tracker*

SLEEP TRACKER:

DATE _____

 RISE: | BEDTIME: | SLEEP (HRS):

NOTES FOR THE DAY

_____

_____

EXERCISE / WORKOUT ROUTINE

IN A STATE OF KETOSIS?

YES   NO   UNSURE

WATER INTAKE TRACKER

DAILY ENERGY LEVEL		
HIGH	**MEDIUM**	**LOW**

BREAKFAST

FAT: CARBS: PROTEIN: CALORIES:

LUNCH

FAT: CARBS: PROTEIN: CALORIES:

DINNER

FAT: CARBS: PROTEIN: CALORIES:

SNACKS

FAT: CARBS: PROTEIN: CALORIES:

TOP 6 PRIORITIES OF THE DAY

END OF THE DAY TOTAL OVERVIEW

CARBS	FAT	PROTEIN	CALORIES

MEAL *Planner*

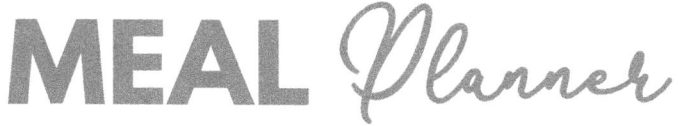

WEEK OF

GROCERY LIST

MON

TUES

WED

THUR

FRI

SAT

SUN

Weekly Meal Planner

Week of: _____

	Breakfast	Lunch	Dinner	Snack	Other
Monday	TOTAL Carbs Fat Protein Cals	TOTAL Carbs Fat Protein Cals	TOTAL Carbs Fat Protein Cals	TOTAL Carbs Fat Protein Cals	TOTAL Carbs Fat Protein Cals
Tuesday	TOTAL Carbs Fat Protein Cals	TOTAL Carbs Fat Protein Cals	TOTAL Carbs Fat Protein Cals	TOTAL Carbs Fat Protein Cals	TOTAL Carbs Fat Protein Cals
Wednesday	TOTAL Carbs Fat Protein Cals	TOTAL Carbs Fat Protein Cals	TOTAL Carbs Fat Protein Cals	TOTAL Carbs Fat Protein Cals	TOTAL Carbs Fat Protein Cals
Thursday	TOTAL Carbs Fat Protein Cals	TOTAL Carbs Fat Protein Cals	TOTAL Carbs Fat Protein Cals	TOTAL Carbs Fat Protein Cals	TOTAL Carbs Fat Protein Cals
Friday	TOTAL Carbs Fat Protein Cals	TOTAL Carbs Fat Protein Cals	TOTAL Carbs Fat Protein Cals	TOTAL Carbs Fat Protein Cals	TOTAL Carbs Fat Protein Cals
Saturday	TOTAL Carbs Fat Protein Cals	TOTAL Carbs Fat Protein Cals	TOTAL Carbs Fat Protein Cals	TOTAL Carbs Fat Protein Cals	TOTAL Carbs Fat Protein Cals
Sunday	TOTAL Carbs Fat Protein Cals	TOTAL Carbs Fat Protein Cals	TOTAL Carbs Fat Protein Cals	TOTAL Carbs Fat Protein Cals	TOTAL Carbs Fat Protein Cals

MY PROGRESS *Tracker*

SLEEP TRACKER:

DATE _____

 RISE: _____

 BEDTIME: _____

 SLEEP (HRS): _____

NOTES FOR THE DAY

_____

_____

_____

IN A STATE OF KETOSIS?

YES   NO   UNSURE

WATER INTAKE TRACKER

EXERCISE / WORKOUT ROUTINE

DAILY ENERGY LEVEL

HIGH	MEDIUM	LOW

BREAKFAST

FAT: CARBS: PROTEIN: CALORIES:

LUNCH

FAT: CARBS: PROTEIN: CALORIES:

DINNER

FAT: CARBS: PROTEIN: CALORIES:

SNACKS

FAT: CARBS: PROTEIN: CALORIES:

TOP 6 PRIORITIES OF THE DAY

END OF THE DAY TOTAL OVERVIEW

CARBS	FAT	PROTEIN	CALORIES

MY PROGRESS *Tracker*

SLEEP TRACKER:

DATE _____

 RISE: _____   BEDTIME: _____   SLEEP (HRS): _____

NOTES FOR THE DAY

_____

_____

_____

IN A STATE OF KETOSIS?

YES   NO   UNSURE

WATER INTAKE TRACKER

EXERCISE / WORKOUT ROUTINE

DAILY ENERGY LEVEL		
HIGH	**MEDIUM**	**LOW**

BREAKFAST

FAT: CARBS: PROTEIN: CALORIES:

LUNCH

FAT: CARBS: PROTEIN: CALORIES:

DINNER

FAT: CARBS: PROTEIN: CALORIES:

SNACKS

FAT: CARBS: PROTEIN: CALORIES:

TOP 6 PRIORITIES OF THE DAY

END OF THE DAY TOTAL OVERVIEW

CARBS   FAT   PROTEIN   CALORIES

MY PROGRESS *Tracker*

SLEEP TRACKER:

DATE _____

 RISE: _____

 BEDTIME: _____

 SLEEP (HRS): _____

NOTES FOR THE DAY

_____

_____

_____

IN A STATE OF KETOSIS?

YES   NO   UNSURE

WATER INTAKE TRACKER

EXERCISE / WORKOUT ROUTINE

DAILY ENERGY LEVEL

HIGH   **MEDIUM**   **LOW**

BREAKFAST

FAT: CARBS: PROTEIN: CALORIES:

LUNCH

FAT: CARBS: PROTEIN: CALORIES:

DINNER

FAT: CARBS: PROTEIN: CALORIES:

SNACKS

FAT: CARBS: PROTEIN: CALORIES:

TOP 6 PRIORITIES OF THE DAY

END OF THE DAY TOTAL OVERVIEW

CARBS   FAT   PROTEIN   CALORIES

MY PROGRESS *Tracker*

SLEEP TRACKER:

☀ RISE: | 🌙 zᶻᶻ BEDTIME: | 💭zᶻᶻ SLEEP (HRS): |

NOTES FOR THE DAY

_____
_____
_____

IN A STATE OF KETOSIS?

YES   NO   UNSURE

WATER INTAKE TRACKER

EXERCISE / WORKOUT ROUTINE

DAILY ENERGY LEVEL		
HIGH	**MEDIUM**	**LOW**

BREAKFAST

FAT: CARBS: PROTEIN: CALORIES:

LUNCH

FAT: CARBS: PROTEIN: CALORIES:

DINNER

FAT: CARBS: PROTEIN: CALORIES:

SNACKS

FAT: CARBS: PROTEIN: CALORIES:

TOP 6 PRIORITIES OF THE DAY

_____
_____

END OF THE DAY TOTAL OVERVIEW

CARBS	FAT	PROTEIN	CALORIES

MY PROGRESS *Tracker*

SLEEP TRACKER:

DATE _____

 RISE: | BEDTIME: | SLEEP (HRS):

NOTES FOR THE DAY

_____

_____

_____

IN A STATE OF KETOSIS?

YES   NO   UNSURE

WATER INTAKE TRACKER

EXERCISE / WORKOUT ROUTINE

DAILY ENERGY LEVEL		
HIGH	**MEDIUM**	**LOW**

BREAKFAST

FAT: CARBS: PROTEIN: CALORIES:

LUNCH

FAT: CARBS: PROTEIN: CALORIES:

DINNER

FAT: CARBS: PROTEIN: CALORIES:

SNACKS

FAT: CARBS: PROTEIN: CALORIES:

TOP 6 PRIORITIES OF THE DAY

END OF THE DAY TOTAL OVERVIEW

CARBS	FAT	PROTEIN	CALORIES

MY PROGRESS *Tracker*

SLEEP TRACKER:

DATE _____

 RISE: _____

 BEDTIME: _____

 SLEEP (HRS): _____

NOTES FOR THE DAY

_____

_____

_____

IN A STATE OF KETOSIS?

YES   NO   UNSURE

WATER INTAKE TRACKER

EXERCISE / WORKOUT ROUTINE

DAILY ENERGY LEVEL		
HIGH	**MEDIUM**	**LOW**

BREAKFAST

FAT: CARBS: PROTEIN: CALORIES:

LUNCH

FAT: CARBS: PROTEIN: CALORIES:

DINNER

FAT: CARBS: PROTEIN: CALORIES:

SNACKS

FAT: CARBS: PROTEIN: CALORIES:

TOP 6 PRIORITIES OF THE DAY

END OF THE DAY TOTAL OVERVIEW

CARBS	FAT	PROTEIN	CALORIES

MY PROGRESS *Tracker*

SLEEP TRACKER:

DATE _____

 RISE: _____   BEDTIME: _____   SLEEP (HRS): _____

NOTES FOR THE DAY

....

....

....

IN A STATE OF KETOSIS?

YES   NO   UNSURE

WATER INTAKE TRACKER

EXERCISE / WORKOUT ROUTINE

DAILY ENERGY LEVEL		
HIGH	**MEDIUM**	**LOW**

BREAKFAST

FAT: CARBS: PROTEIN: CALORIES:

LUNCH

FAT: CARBS: PROTEIN: CALORIES:

DINNER

FAT: CARBS: PROTEIN: CALORIES:

SNACKS

FAT: CARBS: PROTEIN: CALORIES:

TOP 6 PRIORITIES OF THE DAY

END OF THE DAY TOTAL OVERVIEW

CARBS	FAT	PROTEIN	CALORIES

MEAL *Planner*

GROCERY LIST

MON

TUES

WED

THUR

FRI

SAT

SUN

Weekly Meal Planner

Week of:

	Breakfast	Lunch	Dinner	Snack	Other
Monday	TOTAL Carbs Fat Protein Cals	TOTAL Carbs Fat Protein Cals	TOTAL Carbs Fat Protein Cals	TOTAL Carbs Fat Protein Cals	TOTAL Carbs Fat Protein Cals
Tuesday	TOTAL Carbs Fat Protein Cals	TOTAL Carbs Fat Protein Cals	TOTAL Carbs Fat Protein Cals	TOTAL Carbs Fat Protein Cals	TOTAL Carbs Fat Protein Cals
Wednesday	TOTAL Carbs Fat Protein Cals	TOTAL Carbs Fat Protein Cals	TOTAL Carbs Fat Protein Cals	TOTAL Carbs Fat Protein Cals	TOTAL Carbs Fat Protein Cals
Thursday	TOTAL Carbs Fat Protein Cals	TOTAL Carbs Fat Protein Cals	TOTAL Carbs Fat Protein Cals	TOTAL Carbs Fat Protein Cals	TOTAL Carbs Fat Protein Cals
Friday	TOTAL Carbs Fat Protein Cals	TOTAL Carbs Fat Protein Cals	TOTAL Carbs Fat Protein Cals	TOTAL Carbs Fat Protein Cals	TOTAL Carbs Fat Protein Cals
Saturday	TOTAL Carbs Fat Protein Cals	TOTAL Carbs Fat Protein Cals	TOTAL Carbs Fat Protein Cals	TOTAL Carbs Fat Protein Cals	TOTAL Carbs Fat Protein Cals
Sunday	TOTAL Carbs Fat Protein Cals	TOTAL Carbs Fat Protein Cals	TOTAL Carbs Fat Protein Cals	TOTAL Carbs Fat Protein Cals	TOTAL Carbs Fat Protein Cals

MY PROGRESS *Tracker*

SLEEP TRACKER:

 RISE: |_____| BEDTIME: |_____| SLEEP (HRS): |_____|

NOTES FOR THE DAY

_____

_____

_____

IN A STATE OF KETOSIS?

YES   NO   UNSURE

WATER INTAKE TRACKER

EXERCISE / WORKOUT ROUTINE

DAILY ENERGY LEVEL		
HIGH	**MEDIUM**	**LOW**

BREAKFAST

FAT: CARBS: PROTEIN: CALORIES:

LUNCH

FAT: CARBS: PROTEIN: CALORIES:

DINNER

FAT: CARBS: PROTEIN: CALORIES:

SNACKS

FAT: CARBS: PROTEIN: CALORIES:

TOP 6 PRIORITIES OF THE DAY

END OF THE DAY TOTAL OVERVIEW

CARBS   FAT   PROTEIN   CALORIES

_____

_____

MY PROGRESS *Tracker*

SLEEP TRACKER:

DATE _____

 RISE: _____   BEDTIME: _____   SLEEP (HRS): _____

NOTES FOR THE DAY

_____

_____

IN A STATE OF KETOSIS?

YES   NO   UNSURE

WATER INTAKE TRACKER

EXERCISE / WORKOUT ROUTINE

DAILY ENERGY LEVEL		
HIGH	**MEDIUM**	**LOW**

BREAKFAST

FAT: CARBS: PROTEIN: CALORIES:

LUNCH

FAT: CARBS: PROTEIN: CALORIES:

DINNER

FAT: CARBS: PROTEIN: CALORIES:

SNACKS

FAT: CARBS: PROTEIN: CALORIES:

TOP 6 PRIORITIES OF THE DAY

END OF THE DAY TOTAL OVERVIEW

CARBS   FAT   PROTEIN   CALORIES

MY PROGRESS *Tracker*

SLEEP TRACKER:

DATE _____

☀ RISE: _____   🌙 zₖᶻ BEDTIME: _____   ☁zᶻᶻ SLEEP (HRS): _____

NOTES FOR THE DAY

_____
_____
_____

IN A STATE OF KETOSIS?

YES   NO   UNSURE

WATER INTAKE TRACKER

EXERCISE / WORKOUT ROUTINE

DAILY ENERGY LEVEL		
HIGH	**MEDIUM**	**LOW**

BREAKFAST

FAT: CARBS: PROTEIN: CALORIES:

LUNCH

FAT: CARBS: PROTEIN: CALORIES:

DINNER

FAT: CARBS: PROTEIN: CALORIES:

SNACKS

FAT: CARBS: PROTEIN: CALORIES:

TOP 6 PRIORITIES OF THE DAY

END OF THE DAY TOTAL OVERVIEW

CARBS	FAT	PROTEIN	CALORIES

MY PROGRESS *Tracker*

SLEEP TRACKER:

DATE _____

 RISE: _____

 BEDTIME: _____

 SLEEP (HRS): _____

NOTES FOR THE DAY

_____

_____

_____

IN A STATE OF KETOSIS?

YES   NO   UNSURE

WATER INTAKE TRACKER

EXERCISE / WORKOUT ROUTINE

DAILY ENERGY LEVEL		
HIGH	**MEDIUM**	**LOW**

BREAKFAST

FAT: CARBS: PROTEIN: CALORIES:

LUNCH

FAT: CARBS: PROTEIN: CALORIES:

DINNER

FAT: CARBS: PROTEIN: CALORIES:

SNACKS

FAT: CARBS: PROTEIN: CALORIES:

TOP 6 PRIORITIES OF THE DAY

END OF THE DAY TOTAL OVERVIEW

CARBS	FAT	PROTEIN	CALORIES

MY PROGRESS *Tracker*

SLEEP TRACKER:

 RISE: _____

 BEDTIME: _____

 SLEEP (HRS): _____

NOTES FOR THE DAY

_____

_____

_____

IN A STATE OF KETOSIS?

YES   NO   UNSURE

WATER INTAKE TRACKER

EXERCISE / WORKOUT ROUTINE

DAILY ENERGY LEVEL		
HIGH	**MEDIUM**	**LOW**

BREAKFAST

FAT: CARBS: PROTEIN: CALORIES:

LUNCH

FAT: CARBS: PROTEIN: CALORIES:

DINNER

FAT: CARBS: PROTEIN: CALORIES:

SNACKS

FAT: CARBS: PROTEIN: CALORIES:

TOP 6 PRIORITIES OF THE DAY

END OF THE DAY TOTAL OVERVIEW

CARBS	FAT	PROTEIN	CALORIES

MY PROGRESS *Tracker*

SLEEP TRACKER:

DATE _____

 RISE: _____   BEDTIME: _____   SLEEP (HRS): _____

NOTES FOR THE DAY

_____

_____

_____

EXERCISE / WORKOUT ROUTINE

IN A STATE OF KETOSIS?

YES   NO   UNSURE

WATER INTAKE TRACKER

DAILY ENERGY LEVEL		
HIGH	**MEDIUM**	**LOW**

BREAKFAST

FAT: CARBS: PROTEIN: CALORIES:

LUNCH

FAT: CARBS: PROTEIN: CALORIES:

DINNER

FAT: CARBS: PROTEIN: CALORIES:

SNACKS

FAT: CARBS: PROTEIN: CALORIES:

TOP 6 PRIORITIES OF THE DAY

END OF THE DAY TOTAL OVERVIEW

CARBS	FAT	PROTEIN	CALORIES

MY PROGRESS *Tracker*

SLEEP TRACKER:

DATE _____

☀ RISE: | 🌙 zzz BEDTIME: | 💭zZz SLEEP (HRS):

NOTES FOR THE DAY

_____

_____

_____

IN A STATE OF KETOSIS?

YES   NO   UNSURE

WATER INTAKE TRACKER

EXERCISE / WORKOUT ROUTINE

DAILY ENERGY LEVEL		
HIGH	**MEDIUM**	**LOW**

BREAKFAST

FAT: CARBS: PROTEIN: CALORIES:

LUNCH

FAT: CARBS: PROTEIN: CALORIES:

DINNER

FAT: CARBS: PROTEIN: CALORIES:

SNACKS

FAT: CARBS: PROTEIN: CALORIES:

TOP 6 PRIORITIES OF THE DAY

END OF THE DAY TOTAL OVERVIEW

CARBS	FAT	PROTEIN	CALORIES
☐	☐	☐	☐

MEAL 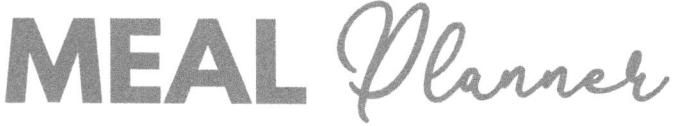 Planner

WEEK OF

GROCERY LIST

MON

TUES

WED

THUR

FRI

SAT

SUN

Weekly Meal Planner

Week of: _____

	Breakfast	Lunch	Dinner	Snack	Other
Monday	TOTAL Carbs Fat Protein Cals	TOTAL Carbs Fat Protein Cals	TOTAL Carbs Fat Protein Cals	TOTAL Carbs Fat Protein Cals	TOTAL Carbs Fat Protein Cals
Tuesday	TOTAL Carbs Fat Protein Cals	TOTAL Carbs Fat Protein Cals	TOTAL Carbs Fat Protein Cals	TOTAL Carbs Fat Protein Cals	TOTAL Carbs Fat Protein Cals
Wednesday	TOTAL Carbs Fat Protein Cals	TOTAL Carbs Fat Protein Cals	TOTAL Carbs Fat Protein Cals	TOTAL Carbs Fat Protein Cals	TOTAL Carbs Fat Protein Cals
Thursday	TOTAL Carbs Fat Protein Cals	TOTAL Carbs Fat Protein Cals	TOTAL Carbs Fat Protein Cals	TOTAL Carbs Fat Protein Cals	TOTAL Carbs Fat Protein Cals
Friday	TOTAL Carbs Fat Protein Cals	TOTAL Carbs Fat Protein Cals	TOTAL Carbs Fat Protein Cals	TOTAL Carbs Fat Protein Cals	TOTAL Carbs Fat Protein Cals
Saturday	TOTAL Carbs Fat Protein Cals	TOTAL Carbs Fat Protein Cals	TOTAL Carbs Fat Protein Cals	TOTAL Carbs Fat Protein Cals	TOTAL Carbs Fat Protein Cals
Sunday	TOTAL Carbs Fat Protein Cals	TOTAL Carbs Fat Protein Cals	TOTAL Carbs Fat Protein Cals	TOTAL Carbs Fat Protein Cals	TOTAL Carbs Fat Protein Cals

MY PROGRESS *Tracker*

SLEEP TRACKER:

DATE _____

 RISE: _____

 BEDTIME: _____

 SLEEP (HRS): _____

NOTES FOR THE DAY

_____

_____

IN A STATE OF KETOSIS?

YES   NO   UNSURE

WATER INTAKE TRACKER

EXERCISE / WORKOUT ROUTINE

DAILY ENERGY LEVEL		
HIGH	**MEDIUM**	**LOW**

BREAKFAST

FAT: CARBS: PROTEIN: CALORIES:

LUNCH

FAT: CARBS: PROTEIN: CALORIES:

DINNER

FAT: CARBS: PROTEIN: CALORIES:

SNACKS

FAT: CARBS: PROTEIN: CALORIES:

TOP 6 PRIORITIES OF THE DAY

END OF THE DAY TOTAL OVERVIEW

CARBS	FAT	PROTEIN	CALORIES

MY PROGRESS *Tracker*

SLEEP TRACKER:

DATE _____

☼ RISE: _____   🌙 zzz BEDTIME: _____   💭zzz SLEEP (HRS): _____

NOTES FOR THE DAY

_____

_____

_____

IN A STATE OF KETOSIS?

YES   NO   UNSURE

WATER INTAKE TRACKER

EXERCISE / WORKOUT ROUTINE

DAILY ENERGY LEVEL		
HIGH	**MEDIUM**	**LOW**

BREAKFAST

FAT: CARBS: PROTEIN: CALORIES:

LUNCH

FAT: CARBS: PROTEIN: CALORIES:

DINNER

FAT: CARBS: PROTEIN: CALORIES:

SNACKS

FAT: CARBS: PROTEIN: CALORIES:

TOP 6 PRIORITIES OF THE DAY

END OF THE DAY TOTAL OVERVIEW

CARBS	FAT	PROTEIN	CALORIES

MY PROGRESS *Tracker*

SLEEP TRACKER:

DATE _____

 RISE: [   ]   BEDTIME: [   ]   SLEEP (HRS): [   ]

NOTES FOR THE DAY

_____

_____

_____

IN A STATE OF KETOSIS?

YES   NO   UNSURE

WATER INTAKE TRACKER

EXERCISE / WORKOUT ROUTINE

DAILY ENERGY LEVEL		
HIGH	**MEDIUM**	**LOW**

BREAKFAST

FAT: CARBS: PROTEIN: CALORIES:

LUNCH

FAT: CARBS: PROTEIN: CALORIES:

DINNER

FAT: CARBS: PROTEIN: CALORIES:

SNACKS

FAT: CARBS: PROTEIN: CALORIES:

TOP 6 PRIORITIES OF THE DAY

END OF THE DAY TOTAL OVERVIEW

CARBS	FAT	PROTEIN	CALORIES

MY PROGRESS *Tracker*

SLEEP TRACKER:

DATE _____

 RISE: [_____]   BEDTIME: [_____]   SLEEP (HRS): [_____]

NOTES FOR THE DAY

_____

_____

IN A STATE OF KETOSIS?

YES   NO   UNSURE

WATER INTAKE TRACKER

EXERCISE / WORKOUT ROUTINE

DAILY ENERGY LEVEL		
HIGH	**MEDIUM**	**LOW**

BREAKFAST

FAT: CARBS: PROTEIN: CALORIES:

LUNCH

FAT: CARBS: PROTEIN: CALORIES:

DINNER

FAT: CARBS: PROTEIN: CALORIES:

SNACKS

FAT: CARBS: PROTEIN: CALORIES:

TOP 6 PRIORITIES OF THE DAY

END OF THE DAY TOTAL OVERVIEW

CARBS	FAT	PROTEIN	CALORIES
[ ]	[ ]	[ ]	[ ]

MY PROGRESS *Tracker*

SLEEP TRACKER:

DATE _____

 RISE: _____   BEDTIME: _____   SLEEP (HRS): _____

NOTES FOR THE DAY

_____

_____

_____

EXERCISE / WORKOUT ROUTINE

IN A STATE OF KETOSIS?

YES   NO   UNSURE

WATER INTAKE TRACKER

DAILY ENERGY LEVEL		
HIGH	**MEDIUM**	**LOW**

BREAKFAST

FAT: CARBS: PROTEIN: CALORIES:

LUNCH

FAT: CARBS: PROTEIN: CALORIES:

DINNER

FAT: CARBS: PROTEIN: CALORIES:

SNACKS

FAT: CARBS: PROTEIN: CALORIES:

TOP 6 PRIORITIES OF THE DAY

END OF THE DAY TOTAL OVERVIEW

CARBS   FAT   PROTEIN   CALORIES

MY PROGRESS *Tracker*

SLEEP TRACKER:

DATE _____

☀ RISE: _____   🌙 z z z BEDTIME: _____   💭 z z z SLEEP (HRS): _____

NOTES FOR THE DAY

_____

_____

_____

IN A STATE OF KETOSIS?

YES   NO   UNSURE

WATER INTAKE TRACKER

EXERCISE / WORKOUT ROUTINE

DAILY ENERGY LEVEL

HIGH	**MEDIUM**	**LOW**

BREAKFAST

FAT: CARBS: PROTEIN: CALORIES:

LUNCH

FAT: CARBS: PROTEIN: CALORIES:

DINNER

FAT: CARBS: PROTEIN: CALORIES:

SNACKS

FAT: CARBS: PROTEIN: CALORIES:

TOP 6 PRIORITIES OF THE DAY

END OF THE DAY TOTAL OVERVIEW

CARBS	FAT	PROTEIN	CALORIES

MY PROGRESS *Tracker*

SLEEP TRACKER:

DATE _____

 RISE: | BEDTIME: | SLEEP (HRS):

NOTES FOR THE DAY

_____
_____
_____

IN A STATE OF KETOSIS?

YES   NO   UNSURE

WATER INTAKE TRACKER

EXERCISE / WORKOUT ROUTINE

DAILY ENERGY LEVEL		
HIGH	**MEDIUM**	**LOW**

BREAKFAST

FAT: CARBS: PROTEIN: CALORIES:

LUNCH

FAT: CARBS: PROTEIN: CALORIES:

DINNER

FAT: CARBS: PROTEIN: CALORIES:

SNACKS

FAT: CARBS: PROTEIN: CALORIES:

TOP 6 PRIORITIES OF THE DAY

_____
_____
_____

END OF THE DAY TOTAL OVERVIEW

CARBS	FAT	PROTEIN	CALORIES

MEAL 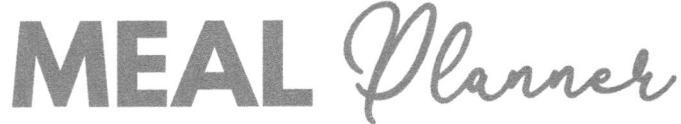 Planner

WEEK OF

GROCERY LIST

MON

TUES

WED

THUR

FRI

SAT

SUN

Weekly Meal Planner

Week of:

	Breakfast	Lunch	Dinner	Snack	Other
Monday	TOTAL Carbs Fat Protein Cals	TOTAL Carbs Fat Protein Cals	TOTAL Carbs Fat Protein Cals	TOTAL Carbs Fat Protein Cals	TOTAL Carbs Fat Protein Cals
Tuesday	TOTAL Carbs Fat Protein Cals	TOTAL Carbs Fat Protein Cals	TOTAL Carbs Fat Protein Cals	TOTAL Carbs Fat Protein Cals	TOTAL Carbs Fat Protein Cals
Wednesday	TOTAL Carbs Fat Protein Cals	TOTAL Carbs Fat Protein Cals	TOTAL Carbs Fat Protein Cals	TOTAL Carbs Fat Protein Cals	TOTAL Carbs Fat Protein Cals
Thursday	TOTAL Carbs Fat Protein Cals	TOTAL Carbs Fat Protein Cals	TOTAL Carbs Fat Protein Cals	TOTAL Carbs Fat Protein Cals	TOTAL Carbs Fat Protein Cals
Friday	TOTAL Carbs Fat Protein Cals	TOTAL Carbs Fat Protein Cals	TOTAL Carbs Fat Protein Cals	TOTAL Carbs Fat Protein Cals	TOTAL Carbs Fat Protein Cals
Saturday	TOTAL Carbs Fat Protein Cals	TOTAL Carbs Fat Protein Cals	TOTAL Carbs Fat Protein Cals	TOTAL Carbs Fat Protein Cals	TOTAL Carbs Fat Protein Cals
Sunday	TOTAL Carbs Fat Protein Cals	TOTAL Carbs Fat Protein Cals	TOTAL Carbs Fat Protein Cals	TOTAL Carbs Fat Protein Cals	TOTAL Carbs Fat Protein Cals

MY PROGRESS *Tracker*

SLEEP TRACKER:

DATE _____

☀ RISE: [ ] 🌙 zzz BEDTIME: [ ] 💭zZz SLEEP (HRS): [ ]

NOTES FOR THE DAY

_____
_____
_____

IN A STATE OF KETOSIS?

YES   NO   UNSURE

WATER INTAKE TRACKER

EXERCISE / WORKOUT ROUTINE

DAILY ENERGY LEVEL		
HIGH	**MEDIUM**	**LOW**

BREAKFAST

FAT: CARBS: PROTEIN: CALORIES:

LUNCH

FAT: CARBS: PROTEIN: CALORIES:

DINNER

FAT: CARBS: PROTEIN: CALORIES:

SNACKS

FAT: CARBS: PROTEIN: CALORIES:

TOP 6 PRIORITIES OF THE DAY

END OF THE DAY TOTAL OVERVIEW

CARBS	FAT	PROTEIN	CALORIES
[ ]	[ ]	[ ]	[ ]

MY PROGRESS *Tracker*

SLEEP TRACKER:

DATE _____

 RISE: _____   BEDTIME: _____   SLEEP (HRS): _____

NOTES FOR THE DAY

_____

_____

_____

IN A STATE OF KETOSIS?

YES   NO   UNSURE

WATER INTAKE TRACKER

EXERCISE / WORKOUT ROUTINE

DAILY ENERGY LEVEL		
HIGH	**MEDIUM**	**LOW**

BREAKFAST

FAT: CARBS: PROTEIN: CALORIES:

LUNCH

FAT: CARBS: PROTEIN: CALORIES:

DINNER

FAT: CARBS: PROTEIN: CALORIES:

SNACKS

FAT: CARBS: PROTEIN: CALORIES:

TOP 6 PRIORITIES OF THE DAY

END OF THE DAY TOTAL OVERVIEW

CARBS	FAT	PROTEIN	CALORIES

MY PROGRESS *Tracker*

SLEEP TRACKER:

 RISE: [   ]   BEDTIME: [   ]   SLEEP (HRS): [   ]

NOTES FOR THE DAY

_____

_____

_____

IN A STATE OF KETOSIS?

YES   NO   UNSURE

WATER INTAKE TRACKER

EXERCISE / WORKOUT ROUTINE

DAILY ENERGY LEVEL		
HIGH	**MEDIUM**	**LOW**

BREAKFAST

FAT: CARBS: PROTEIN: CALORIES:

LUNCH

FAT: CARBS: PROTEIN: CALORIES:

DINNER

FAT: CARBS: PROTEIN: CALORIES:

SNACKS

FAT: CARBS: PROTEIN: CALORIES:

TOP 6 PRIORITIES OF THE DAY

_____

_____

END OF THE DAY TOTAL OVERVIEW

CARBS	FAT	PROTEIN	CALORIES
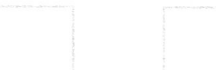			

MY PROGRESS *Tracker*

SLEEP TRACKER:

DATE _____

 RISE: _____   BEDTIME: _____   SLEEP (HRS): _____

NOTES FOR THE DAY

_____

_____

IN A STATE OF KETOSIS?

YES   NO   UNSURE

WATER INTAKE TRACKER

EXERCISE / WORKOUT ROUTINE

DAILY ENERGY LEVEL		
HIGH	**MEDIUM**	**LOW**

BREAKFAST

FAT: CARBS: PROTEIN: CALORIES:

LUNCH

FAT: CARBS: PROTEIN: CALORIES:

DINNER

FAT: CARBS: PROTEIN: CALORIES:

SNACKS

FAT: CARBS: PROTEIN: CALORIES:

TOP 6 PRIORITIES OF THE DAY

END OF THE DAY TOTAL OVERVIEW

CARBS   FAT   PROTEIN   CALORIES

MY PROGRESS *Tracker*

SLEEP TRACKER:

DATE _____

RISE: _____   BEDTIME: _____   SLEEP (HRS): _____

NOTES FOR THE DAY

_____
_____
_____

IN A STATE OF KETOSIS?

YES   NO   UNSURE

WATER INTAKE TRACKER

EXERCISE / WORKOUT ROUTINE

DAILY ENERGY LEVEL		
HIGH	**MEDIUM**	**LOW**

BREAKFAST

FAT: CARBS: PROTEIN: CALORIES:

LUNCH

FAT: CARBS: PROTEIN: CALORIES:

DINNER

FAT: CARBS: PROTEIN: CALORIES:

SNACKS

FAT: CARBS: PROTEIN: CALORIES:

TOP 6 PRIORITIES OF THE DAY

END OF THE DAY TOTAL OVERVIEW

CARBS	FAT	PROTEIN	CALORIES

MY PROGRESS *Tracker*

SLEEP TRACKER:

DATE _____

 RISE: _____   BEDTIME: _____   SLEEP (HRS): _____

NOTES FOR THE DAY

_____

_____

_____

IN A STATE OF KETOSIS?

YES   NO   UNSURE

WATER INTAKE TRACKER

EXERCISE / WORKOUT ROUTINE

DAILY ENERGY LEVEL		
HIGH	**MEDIUM**	**LOW**

BREAKFAST

FAT: CARBS: PROTEIN: CALORIES:

LUNCH

FAT: CARBS: PROTEIN: CALORIES:

DINNER

FAT: CARBS: PROTEIN: CALORIES:

SNACKS

FAT: CARBS: PROTEIN: CALORIES:

TOP 6 PRIORITIES OF THE DAY

END OF THE DAY TOTAL OVERVIEW

CARBS	FAT	PROTEIN	CALORIES

MY PROGRESS *Tracker*

SLEEP TRACKER:

DATE _____

 RISE: _____   BEDTIME: _____   SLEEP (HRS): _____

NOTES FOR THE DAY

_____

_____

_____

IN A STATE OF KETOSIS?

YES   NO   UNSURE

WATER INTAKE TRACKER

EXERCISE / WORKOUT ROUTINE

DAILY ENERGY LEVEL		
HIGH	**MEDIUM**	**LOW**

BREAKFAST

FAT: CARBS: PROTEIN: CALORIES:

LUNCH

FAT: CARBS: PROTEIN: CALORIES:

DINNER

FAT: CARBS: PROTEIN: CALORIES:

SNACKS

FAT: CARBS: PROTEIN: CALORIES:

TOP 6 PRIORITIES OF THE DAY

END OF THE DAY TOTAL OVERVIEW

CARBS   FAT   PROTEIN   CALORIES

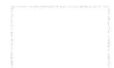   

MEAL *Planner*

WEEK OF

GROCERY LIST

MON

TUES

WED

THUR

FRI

SAT

SUN

Weekly Meal Planner

Week of: _____

	Breakfast	Lunch	Dinner	Snack	Other
Monday	TOTAL Carbs Fat Protein Cals	TOTAL Carbs Fat Protein Cals	TOTAL Carbs Fat Protein Cals	TOTAL Carbs Fat Protein Cals	TOTAL Carbs Fat Protein Cals
Tuesday	TOTAL Carbs Fat Protein Cals	TOTAL Carbs Fat Protein Cals	TOTAL Carbs Fat Protein Cals	TOTAL Carbs Fat Protein Cals	TOTAL Carbs Fat Protein Cals
Wednesday	TOTAL Carbs Fat Protein Cals	TOTAL Carbs Fat Protein Cals	TOTAL Carbs Fat Protein Cals	TOTAL Carbs Fat Protein Cals	TOTAL Carbs Fat Protein Cals
Thursday	TOTAL Carbs Fat Protein Cals	TOTAL Carbs Fat Protein Cals	TOTAL Carbs Fat Protein Cals	TOTAL Carbs Fat Protein Cals	TOTAL Carbs Fat Protein Cals
Friday	TOTAL Carbs Fat Protein Cals	TOTAL Carbs Fat Protein Cals	TOTAL Carbs Fat Protein Cals	TOTAL Carbs Fat Protein Cals	TOTAL Carbs Fat Protein Cals
Saturday	TOTAL Carbs Fat Protein Cals	TOTAL Carbs Fat Protein Cals	TOTAL Carbs Fat Protein Cals	TOTAL Carbs Fat Protein Cals	TOTAL Carbs Fat Protein Cals
Sunday	TOTAL Carbs Fat Protein Cals	TOTAL Carbs Fat Protein Cals	TOTAL Carbs Fat Protein Cals	TOTAL Carbs Fat Protein Cals	TOTAL Carbs Fat Protein Cals

MY PROGRESS *Tracker*

SLEEP TRACKER:

DATE _____

 RISE: _____

 BEDTIME: _____

 SLEEP (HRS): _____

NOTES FOR THE DAY

_____
_____
_____

EXERCISE / WORKOUT ROUTINE

IN A STATE OF KETOSIS?

YES   NO   UNSURE

WATER INTAKE TRACKER

DAILY ENERGY LEVEL		
HIGH	**MEDIUM**	**LOW**

BREAKFAST

FAT: CARBS: PROTEIN: CALORIES:

LUNCH

FAT: CARBS: PROTEIN: CALORIES:

DINNER

FAT: CARBS: PROTEIN: CALORIES:

SNACKS

FAT: CARBS: PROTEIN: CALORIES:

TOP 6 PRIORITIES OF THE DAY

END OF THE DAY TOTAL OVERVIEW

CARBS	FAT	PROTEIN	CALORIES

MY PROGRESS *Tracker*

SLEEP TRACKER:

 RISE: BEDTIME: SLEEP (HRS):

DATE _____

NOTES FOR THE DAY

_____

_____

IN A STATE OF KETOSIS?

YES   NO   UNSURE

WATER INTAKE TRACKER

EXERCISE / WORKOUT ROUTINE

DAILY ENERGY LEVEL		
HIGH	**MEDIUM**	**LOW**

BREAKFAST

FAT: CARBS: PROTEIN: CALORIES:

LUNCH

FAT: CARBS: PROTEIN: CALORIES:

DINNER

FAT: CARBS: PROTEIN: CALORIES:

SNACKS

FAT: CARBS: PROTEIN: CALORIES:

TOP 6 PRIORITIES OF THE DAY

END OF THE DAY TOTAL OVERVIEW

CARBS	FAT	PROTEIN	CALORIES

MY PROGRESS *Tracker*

SLEEP TRACKER:

 RISE: _____

 BEDTIME: _____

DATE _____

 SLEEP (HRS): _____

NOTES FOR THE DAY

_____

_____

IN A STATE OF KETOSIS?

YES   NO   UNSURE

WATER INTAKE TRACKER

EXERCISE / WORKOUT ROUTINE

DAILY ENERGY LEVEL		
HIGH	**MEDIUM**	**LOW**

BREAKFAST

FAT: CARBS: PROTEIN: CALORIES:

LUNCH

FAT: CARBS: PROTEIN: CALORIES:

DINNER

FAT: CARBS: PROTEIN: CALORIES:

SNACKS

FAT: CARBS: PROTEIN: CALORIES:

TOP 6 PRIORITIES OF THE DAY

END OF THE DAY TOTAL OVERVIEW

CARBS	FAT	PROTEIN	CALORIES

MY PROGRESS *Tracker*

SLEEP TRACKER:

 RISE: BEDTIME: SLEEP (HRS):

DATE _____

NOTES FOR THE DAY

_____

_____

_____

EXERCISE / WORKOUT ROUTINE

IN A STATE OF KETOSIS?

YES   NO   UNSURE

WATER INTAKE TRACKER

DAILY ENERGY LEVEL		
HIGH	**MEDIUM**	**LOW**

BREAKFAST

FAT: CARBS: PROTEIN: CALORIES:

LUNCH

FAT: CARBS: PROTEIN: CALORIES:

DINNER

FAT: CARBS: PROTEIN: CALORIES:

SNACKS

FAT: CARBS: PROTEIN: CALORIES:

TOP 6 PRIORITIES OF THE DAY

END OF THE DAY TOTAL OVERVIEW

CARBS	FAT	PROTEIN	CALORIES

MY PROGRESS *Tracker*

SLEEP TRACKER:

DATE _____

 RISE: | BEDTIME: | SLEEP (HRS):

NOTES FOR THE DAY

_____

_____

_____

IN A STATE OF KETOSIS?

YES   NO   UNSURE

WATER INTAKE TRACKER

EXERCISE / WORKOUT ROUTINE

DAILY ENERGY LEVEL		
HIGH	**MEDIUM**	**LOW**

BREAKFAST

FAT: CARBS: PROTEIN: CALORIES:

LUNCH

FAT: CARBS: PROTEIN: CALORIES:

DINNER

FAT: CARBS: PROTEIN: CALORIES:

SNACKS

FAT: CARBS: PROTEIN: CALORIES:

TOP 6 PRIORITIES OF THE DAY

END OF THE DAY TOTAL OVERVIEW

CARBS   FAT   PROTEIN   CALORIES

MY PROGRESS *Tracker*

SLEEP TRACKER:

DATE _____

 RISE: _____   BEDTIME: _____   SLEEP (HRS): _____

NOTES FOR THE DAY

_____

_____

_____

EXERCISE / WORKOUT ROUTINE

IN A STATE OF KETOSIS?

YES   NO   UNSURE

WATER INTAKE TRACKER

DAILY ENERGY LEVEL		
HIGH	**MEDIUM**	**LOW**

BREAKFAST

FAT: CARBS: PROTEIN: CALORIES:

LUNCH

FAT: CARBS: PROTEIN: CALORIES:

DINNER

FAT: CARBS: PROTEIN: CALORIES:

SNACKS

FAT: CARBS: PROTEIN: CALORIES:

TOP 6 PRIORITIES OF THE DAY

_____

_____

END OF THE DAY TOTAL OVERVIEW

CARBS	FAT	PROTEIN	CALORIES

MY PROGRESS *Tracker*

SLEEP TRACKER:

DATE _____

 RISE: _____

 BEDTIME: _____

 SLEEP (HRS): _____

NOTES FOR THE DAY

_____
_____

IN A STATE OF KETOSIS?

YES   NO   UNSURE

WATER INTAKE TRACKER

EXERCISE / WORKOUT ROUTINE

DAILY ENERGY LEVEL		
HIGH	**MEDIUM**	**LOW**

BREAKFAST

FAT: CARBS: PROTEIN: CALORIES:

LUNCH

FAT: CARBS: PROTEIN: CALORIES:

DINNER

FAT: CARBS: PROTEIN: CALORIES:

SNACKS

FAT: CARBS: PROTEIN: CALORIES:

TOP 6 PRIORITIES OF THE DAY

END OF THE DAY TOTAL OVERVIEW

CARBS   FAT   PROTEIN   CALORIES

MEAL 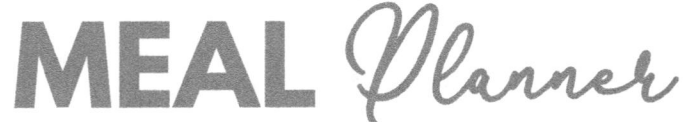 Planner

WEEK OF

GROCERY LIST

MON

TUES

WED

THUR

FRI

SAT

SUN

Weekly Meal Planner

Week of: _____

	Breakfast	Lunch	Dinner	Snack	Other
Monday	TOTAL Carbs Fat Protein Cals	TOTAL Carbs Fat Protein Cals	TOTAL Carbs Fat Protein Cals	TOTAL Carbs Fat Protein Cals	TOTAL Carbs Fat Protein Cals
Tuesday	TOTAL Carbs Fat Protein Cals	TOTAL Carbs Fat Protein Cals	TOTAL Carbs Fat Protein Cals	TOTAL Carbs Fat Protein Cals	TOTAL Carbs Fat Protein Cals
Wednesday	TOTAL Carbs Fat Protein Cals	TOTAL Carbs Fat Protein Cals	TOTAL Carbs Fat Protein Cals	TOTAL Carbs Fat Protein Cals	TOTAL Carbs Fat Protein Cals
Thursday	TOTAL Carbs Fat Protein Cals	TOTAL Carbs Fat Protein Cals	TOTAL Carbs Fat Protein Cals	TOTAL Carbs Fat Protein Cals	TOTAL Carbs Fat Protein Cals
Friday	TOTAL Carbs Fat Protein Cals	TOTAL Carbs Fat Protein Cals	TOTAL Carbs Fat Protein Cals	TOTAL Carbs Fat Protein Cals	TOTAL Carbs Fat Protein Cals
Saturday	TOTAL Carbs Fat Protein Cals	TOTAL Carbs Fat Protein Cals	TOTAL Carbs Fat Protein Cals	TOTAL Carbs Fat Protein Cals	TOTAL Carbs Fat Protein Cals
Sunday	TOTAL Carbs Fat Protein Cals	TOTAL Carbs Fat Protein Cals	TOTAL Carbs Fat Protein Cals	TOTAL Carbs Fat Protein Cals	TOTAL Carbs Fat Protein Cals

MY PROGRESS *Tracker*

SLEEP TRACKER:

 RISE: BEDTIME: SLEEP (HRS):

DATE _____

NOTES FOR THE DAY

_____

_____

_____

IN A STATE OF KETOSIS?

YES   NO   UNSURE

WATER INTAKE TRACKER

EXERCISE / WORKOUT ROUTINE

DAILY ENERGY LEVEL		
HIGH	**MEDIUM**	**LOW**

BREAKFAST

FAT: CARBS: PROTEIN: CALORIES:

LUNCH

FAT: CARBS: PROTEIN: CALORIES:

DINNER

FAT: CARBS: PROTEIN: CALORIES:

SNACKS

FAT: CARBS: PROTEIN: CALORIES:

TOP 6 PRIORITIES OF THE DAY

END OF THE DAY TOTAL OVERVIEW

CARBS	FAT	PROTEIN	CALORIES

MY PROGRESS *Tracker*

SLEEP TRACKER:

DATE _____

 RISE: |_____| BEDTIME: |_____| SLEEP (HRS): |_____|

NOTES FOR THE DAY

_____

_____

_____

EXERCISE / WORKOUT ROUTINE

IN A STATE OF KETOSIS?

YES   NO   UNSURE

WATER INTAKE TRACKER

DAILY ENERGY LEVEL		
HIGH	**MEDIUM**	**LOW**

BREAKFAST

FAT: CARBS: PROTEIN: CALORIES:

LUNCH

FAT: CARBS: PROTEIN: CALORIES:

DINNER

FAT: CARBS: PROTEIN: CALORIES:

SNACKS

FAT: CARBS: PROTEIN: CALORIES:

TOP 6 PRIORITIES OF THE DAY

END OF THE DAY TOTAL OVERVIEW

CARBS	FAT	PROTEIN	CALORIES

MY PROGRESS *Tracker*

SLEEP TRACKER:

DATE _____

☀ RISE: _____   🌙 z_z_z BEDTIME: _____   💭 zᶻz SLEEP (HRS): _____

NOTES FOR THE DAY

_____

_____

_____

IN A STATE OF KETOSIS?

YES   NO   UNSURE

WATER INTAKE TRACKER

EXERCISE / WORKOUT ROUTINE

DAILY ENERGY LEVEL		
HIGH	**MEDIUM**	**LOW**

BREAKFAST

FAT: CARBS: PROTEIN: CALORIES:

LUNCH

FAT: CARBS: PROTEIN: CALORIES:

DINNER

FAT: CARBS: PROTEIN: CALORIES:

SNACKS

FAT: CARBS: PROTEIN: CALORIES:

TOP 6 PRIORITIES OF THE DAY

_____

_____

END OF THE DAY TOTAL OVERVIEW

CARBS   FAT   PROTEIN   CALORIES

MY PROGRESS *Tracker*

SLEEP TRACKER:

DATE _____

 RISE: | BEDTIME: | SLEEP (HRS):

NOTES FOR THE DAY

_____
_____
_____

IN A STATE OF KETOSIS?

YES   NO   UNSURE

WATER INTAKE TRACKER

EXERCISE / WORKOUT ROUTINE

DAILY ENERGY LEVEL		
HIGH	**MEDIUM**	**LOW**

BREAKFAST

FAT: CARBS: PROTEIN: CALORIES:

LUNCH

FAT: CARBS: PROTEIN: CALORIES:

DINNER

FAT: CARBS: PROTEIN: CALORIES:

SNACKS

FAT: CARBS: PROTEIN: CALORIES:

TOP 6 PRIORITIES OF THE DAY

END OF THE DAY TOTAL OVERVIEW

CARBS   FAT   PROTEIN   CALORIES

MY PROGRESS *Tracker*

SLEEP TRACKER:

DATE _____

 RISE: _____   BEDTIME: _____   SLEEP (HRS): _____

NOTES FOR THE DAY

_____

_____

_____

IN A STATE OF KETOSIS?

YES   NO   UNSURE

WATER INTAKE TRACKER

EXERCISE / WORKOUT ROUTINE

DAILY ENERGY LEVEL		
HIGH	**MEDIUM**	**LOW**

BREAKFAST

FAT: CARBS: PROTEIN: CALORIES:

LUNCH

FAT: CARBS: PROTEIN: CALORIES:

DINNER

FAT: CARBS: PROTEIN: CALORIES:

SNACKS

FAT: CARBS: PROTEIN: CALORIES:

TOP 6 PRIORITIES OF THE DAY

END OF THE DAY TOTAL OVERVIEW

CARBS	FAT	PROTEIN	CALORIES

MY PROGRESS *Tracker*

SLEEP TRACKER:

DATE _____

 RISE: _____   BEDTIME: _____   SLEEP (HRS): _____

NOTES FOR THE DAY

_____

_____

_____

EXERCISE / WORKOUT ROUTINE

IN A STATE OF KETOSIS?

YES   NO   UNSURE

WATER INTAKE TRACKER

DAILY ENERGY LEVEL		
HIGH	**MEDIUM**	**LOW**

BREAKFAST

FAT: CARBS: PROTEIN: CALORIES:

LUNCH

FAT: CARBS: PROTEIN: CALORIES:

DINNER

FAT: CARBS: PROTEIN: CALORIES:

SNACKS

FAT: CARBS: PROTEIN: CALORIES:

TOP 6 PRIORITIES OF THE DAY

END OF THE DAY TOTAL OVERVIEW

CARBS   FAT   PROTEIN   CALORIES

MY PROGRESS *Tracker*

SLEEP TRACKER:

DATE _____

☀ RISE: _____   🌙 zzz BEDTIME: _____   💭zᶻᶻ SLEEP (HRS): _____

NOTES FOR THE DAY

_____
_____
_____

IN A STATE OF KETOSIS?

YES   NO   UNSURE

WATER INTAKE TRACKER

EXERCISE / WORKOUT ROUTINE

DAILY ENERGY LEVEL		
HIGH	**MEDIUM**	**LOW**

BREAKFAST

FAT: CARBS: PROTEIN: CALORIES:

LUNCH

FAT: CARBS: PROTEIN: CALORIES:

DINNER

FAT: CARBS: PROTEIN: CALORIES:

SNACKS

FAT: CARBS: PROTEIN: CALORIES:

TOP 6 PRIORITIES OF THE DAY

_____
_____

END OF THE DAY TOTAL OVERVIEW

CARBS	FAT	PROTEIN	CALORIES